# pregnancy & childbirth

## SECRETS

### GAIL J. DAHL

**Innovative Publishing**

Published by Innovative Publishing

http://web.mac.com/pregnancysecrets

Cover Design by Clean Line Design
Printed by Transcontinental Printing
Index by Clive Pyne Book Indexing Services

Distributed by: Gordon Soules Book Publishers Ltd.
1359 Ambleside Lane, West Vancouver, BC, Canada  V7T 2Y9
(604) 922-6588 or (604) 688-5466 Fax: (604) 688-5442
E-mail: books@gordonsoules.com

Reduction of ecological footprint using Regeneration-100 instead of virgin fibers paper reduces the ecological footprint of 42 trees, 2,684 pounds of solid waste, 25,337 gallons of water, 17.0 pounds of suspended particles in water, 5,895 pounds of air emissions and 6,143 cubic feet of natural gas.

Library and Archives Cataloguing in Publication
Dahl, Gail J
Pregnancy & Childbirth Secrets / Gail J. Dahl.
Includes bibliographical references and index.
ISBN 978-1-896937-08-3
1. Pregnancy--Popular works. 2. Childbirth--Popular works. 3. Newborn
infants--Care. I. Title. II. Title: Pregnancy and Childbirth Secrets.

Printed in Canada on Recycled Paper
10 9 8 7 6 5 3 4 2 1 2009 2008 2007

*This book is dedicated to my daughter, Sabrina;*
*my anchor and inspiration.*

# Table of Contents

# **Foreword**

Pregnancy and childbirth are pivotal life events. At these times, we witness and experience the indescribable miracle of new life unfolding within us and before us. More real than any nature documentary -- and more confronting at times -- this extraordinary process happens within our most intimate spaces: our body, our home, our family.

The details of these events, and the emotions surrounding them, will be etched on our minds and bodies for life. When they are positive experiences, we can gain the deep joy and unshakeable confidence that will sustain us through not only the intense newborn days, but also the months and years that follow.

Such a positive start is no accident or unrealistic dream: it is what Mother Nature prescribes for all of us. Beginning in early pregnancy every woman's body produces, in increasing amounts, a cocktail of hormones-- natural body chemicals -- that help to create an ideal situation for our baby's growth and development. These include oxytocin, the love hormone; beta-endorphin, hormone of pleasure; epinephrine/norepinephrine (adrenaline/noradrenalin) hormones of excitement, and prolactin, hormone of tenderness. In pregnancy, these hormones, released from the limbic system or emotional brain, enhance the expectant mother's digestion and nutrition, and help her to remain calm and connected with her growing baby.

In labor, levels of these hormones increase further, supporting the laboring woman's mind and body. Physically they are responsible for some of the actual processes of labor and birth, and help to maximize safety for mother and baby. Emotionally, they imprint an ecstatic cocktail of love, pleasure, excitement and tenderness. Levels of the ecstatic hormones peak in the hour or so after birth so that both mother and baby are in an ideal hormonal balance at first meeting, ecstatic and primed to begin their new relationship with joy and confidence.

This ideal beginning is unfortunately much less likely when there is medical intervention in labor. Many of the most common interventions, such as inductions, epidurals, spinals and cesareans will interfere with the delicate orchestration of these ecstatic hormones. This can make birth more difficult, and even less safe, for both mother and baby.

In these circumstances, the natural feelings of joy and confidence after birth may be replaced by disappointment and fear, and the feeling that our bodies have failed us. We may lose our bearings, and the start will likely be harder for all the family. Sometimes we need to accept that such intervention was necessary for the well-being of mother or baby. However for the vast majority, birth will proceed most easily and safely with the emphasis on privacy and sensitive support rather than continual observations and medical procedures.

How can we maximize our chances of ease, pleasure and safety at birth? How can we minimize our need for interventions? Can we begin, even from early pregnancy, to increase our poise and self-possession, and take the steps that are most likely to give us a joyful and confident start?

Fortunately, this journey -- the journey towards natural birth --is mapped out here before you. Gail Dahl has assembled a treasure-trove of wisdom from some of the foremost experts in the area. Not only is there wisdom and experience, but she includes the scientific evidence that you need, presented in easily understandable language. And, like a good friend, Pregnancy and Childbirth Secrets is with you through the whole journey and comes in with just the information and advice that you need at the right time.

Pregnancy and childbirth are pivotal life events. Pregnancy and Childbirth Secrets will give you the resources you need for a gentle, joyful, and confident start for your whole family.

Dr. Sarah J. Buckley, GP/Family Physician, author of Gentle Birth, Gentle Mothering – The Wisdom and Science of Gentle Choices in Pregnancy, Birth and Parenting.

# Introduction

As I began the journey of bringing in a new life into the world, I searched for information to move safely to this next destination. I remember throwing the last book I read across the room, wondering: "Why is it so difficult to find out what really happens during childbirth? In the past one hundred years haven't we learned anything more about childbirth than breathing in rhythm? Why is it all such a secret?"

Most books on the market dealt thoroughly with pregnancy, which women are very good at, with only a few pages at the back of the book on childbirth. The few pages remaining showed a diagram of a woman with half her body removed. There were more books available on naming a baby that on having one. It seemed there was very little time to accumulate the answers to these important questions. Even though I was able to take advantage of prenatal appointments and prenatal classes, the questions still remained.

During the birth of my daughter, I had both good and bad experiences. Shortly after her birth, I felt moved to stop and record what I had learned about pregnancy and childbirth so that I could pass this valuable knowledge on to my daughter. When I had recorded everything I had learned, I began to think about the other mothers. What about the mother who had three children, four children, and what about the mother who had experienced six or more births? What did that mother know about childbirth? I felt each mother held a portion of the key that could unlock the secrets of childbirth. Perhaps what was needed was to collect all this accumulated wisdom into one place. In addition, I began to research exactly what had gone wrong during the birth of my own daughter.

What I didn't know when I placed my first newspaper advertisement asking mothers to call in with their best tips on pregnancy, childbirth, breastfeeding and newborn care was that I would be setting off a virtual political powder keg where each interest group declared they, and they alone, held the key to the secrets to childbirth.

My phone began to ring off the hook within twenty-four hours of running the advertisements and didn't stop until years afterward. Some of the childbirth stories I heard were heartbreaking; some were the absolute opposite and left me feeling completely uplifted. A common theme, however, was that women the world over were looking for a means to tell their birth story and, in turn, a way to help other mothers and daughters with their childbirth experiences. The encouragement for me to write about birth from a woman's viewpoint was overwhelming. Each telephone call and written survey I received moved me deeper into the field of childbirth.

Some of the mothers I interviewed had very difficult birth experiences and wanted to pass this information on so that other women would not have to go through what they had. Other mothers had planned, positive childbirth experiences and wanted new mothers to share what they had discovered from childbirth. Fathers called in to help other new fathers with their responsibilities in the labor and delivery rooms. I began to interview medical professionals for their opinions and knowledge regarding childbirth.

I continued this research by working with some of the world's greatest childbirth experts, asking for contributions of research articles that could vastly improve the health of mothers and babies. In the end, I achieved an incredible overview of the process of childbirth with secrets collected from both sides.

What surprised me most during this process was to find out that many of today's common medical interventions are often unnecessary. For instance, any of the following common medical practices can cause a woman's labor to be more painful and prolonged, and the baby's delivery more difficult: having to labor on your back; endless mechanical monitoring of the baby; IV's; being unable to eat or drink during labor; restricting physical activity; and routinely using drugs to force or speed up labor. Each of these medical procedures can trigger a cascade of additional unwanted medical interventions from which there may be no safe return. Each additional technological intervention puts mother and baby at further risk during childbirth.

I became aware of the damages that were being done by the medicalized births our society has created. Some women felt emotionally traumatized during the birth of their babies. Some women who had been induced reported a feeling of being "raped" of their babies, rather than birthing them. Then there were some mothers who, not yet recovered from a traumatic birth experience, were physically or emotionally unable to add to their families before their biological clock ran out.

Many mothers have had to deal with prolonged postnatal depression caused by traumatic childbirth and induction drugs. Secondary infertility caused by cesarean birth has left mothers unable to have additional children. A violent or traumatic birth, combined with prolonged postnatal depression, can erode a good relationship between mother and father and may lead to separation or divorce. A mother who has had a difficult birth experience may find it hard to bond with her baby causing great difficulties in the relationship between mother and child throughout the formative years.

A baby exposed to a large number of drugs during a traumatic birth will have difficulty breastfeeding due to the afterlife of these powerful drugs in their small bodies. Worse still, babies who experience a "drugged high" at birth may be at greater risk of developing chemical addictions later in life. Babies routinely taken away from the mother in the first hours of birth cause intense stress hormones to be released in the baby. The mother's production of parenting hormones can be arrested or stopped completely if her baby is taken away during the first few hours after the birth. The mother needs these hours immediately after childbirth to see, smell and touch her baby in order to release the natural parenting hormones within her body. The baby needs to breastfeed immediately after the birth in order to take advantage of instinctual breastfeeding.

Intense medical intervention in the birth of your baby may also cause a lack of oxygen which can cause permanent brain damage or learning disabilities in your baby. Induced babies may suffer head injuries during birth, from pounding on an incomplete pelvic floor which can lead to crying baby syndrome for months afterwards, thereby creating havoc within the new family unit. Our obstetricians do not see any of this fallout that occurs with today's medicalized births as the aftercare of babies and mothers is passed on to the family doctor and the pediatrician.

Ever increasing use of induction drugs achieves daytime deliveries, but at what cost to the our families and our future society? These are just some of the more devastating outcomes to our new families created by what has become a "faster is better" managed birth culture in North America.

So, how is this chain of events allowed to take place? It usually begins with a physician or a midwife saying: "I'm going to give you a little something to get you going." This seemingly minor medical intervention can cause a cascade of increasingly more serious medical interventions that quickly follow this decision.

The initial decision to get the mother "going" will cause her to become swamped with wave after wave of forced, mechanical contractions, created by the birth induction drugs. The mother may then ask for something to help her with the pain, even if she has sworn not to take drugs during childbirth. Pain medication follows to counteract the unnatural pain of these forced, artificial contractions.

Now, because of the recently administered pain drugs the mother's artificial labor will likely slow or completely stop. At this point, further induction drugs are required to get the drugged, artificial labor contractions back on track.

It is common at this time for the baby to go into distress. This is caused by induction and pain medications, which can trigger a reduced supply of oxygen to the baby. Because the contractions are forced and unnatural, the baby may be unable to catch its breath. In addition, the pain medication is too strong for the baby's tiny body and may cause the baby to be unable to move into a good birth position, further restricting the supply of oxygen. The mother is often lying unnaturally on her back which can also compromise the supply of oxygen to her baby.

Now the fetal distress is real and must be dealt with immediately. By attempting to "schedule" birth, a medical emergency has been created. Because of the real danger of brain damage due to lack of oxygen, the baby may now have to be delivered forcibly through additional medical interventions such as vacuum or forceps delivery with episiotomy, both of which present the potential for brain damage to the infant and physical trauma to the mother.

If these additional interventions fail, the last possible birth medical intervention card must be played with the mother and baby taken away for an emergency cesarean section.

Many parents have been swept up in this scenario by agreeing to "a little something", to induce labor, without fully understanding what this decision entails. The existing prenatal education system is no more than a hit-and-miss proposition offering very little practical information to the small percentage of new parents lucky or wealthy enough to partake of it. Most existing prenatal classes teach women to be good patients. With resources limited, physicians often don't have time to explain each procedure and the associated risks to each expectant parent.

As men have taken over managing birth, they are unable to experience the difference in the increased pain levels of a forced or artificial labor and a normal labor. As men do not experience labor they don't realize that they are "over helping" women with extremely strong pain relief causing labors to be longer than they would normally have to be. By managing birth they are creating a mismanagement in the natural order of what birth is supposed to be, bypassing a woman's own innate ability to safely and effectively deal with the rigors of childbirth.

By inducing birth, more and more babies are being born prematurely not giving the baby enough time for the final development of their lungs and other last finishing touches that occur within the womb in the last days of development and as the mother begins to labor when her body and baby are ready.

I began to see that the women with the best childbirth experiences had done their homework. They had hired independent professionals to assist them with the birthing process, regardless of where they chose to give birth: at a hospital, birthing center or a quiet home setting. These women had created a calm, gentle and undisturbed birth environment wherever they were. They could walk about or shift positioning during labor. They had access to warm water in the form of showers or bathtubs. They had massages, and food and drink available to refresh them during the labor process, and there was constant coaching and a constant presence given to both mother and father by the birthing professionals. These were some of their secrets to having a safe and gentle birth experience. These births started naturally at the exact time both the mother's body and the baby were ready, and continued naturally, their labors were less painful and shorter, delivering the baby was less painful and of a shorter duration leaving both mother and baby able to recover more quickly from the emotional and physical effects of childbirth.

I began to realize that perhaps the secret to childbirth includes educating mothers- and fathers-to-be before a pregnancy occurs. Pregnancy, childbirth, breastfeeding and newborn care information are basic to our society's health and need to be treated as such within our school system. Education is the only way to dissipate the unnecessary fear surrounding childbirth. It is time that women of every economic and educational level are given the tools to understand how their bodies work during pregnancy, childbirth and beyond, and what can be done to create a better birth experience. By educating both men and women about childbirth, rather than the rare few, we can make a significant difference in the lives of our future families. Research shows that women make better decisions in regard to childbirth when they are fully informed.

It was a surprise when I discovered many of our doctors and nurses had opted out of our traditional hospital birthing system and were turning to birthing centers or quiet births at home for their families. This growing number of doctors and nurses were looking for a different childbirth experience and they were finding it.

Gentle birth advocates create a positive, planned childbirth partnered with professional labor support and reap the rewards of an empowering childbirth experience. These mothers experience a faster physical recovery from childbirth with little or no emotional difficulties; the fathers feel more involved in the childbirth experience with less pressure to know everything; the babies are healthier, calmer and bond more readily with both parents. A healthier and happier mother and baby is what these birth advocates are after. A gentle, safe and undisturbed birth will give the best results for the entire family.

Mounting evidence shows that each needless birth intervention puts mother and baby at an ever-increasing risk of complication. Take the time to investigate the risks that some of these new medical interventions can have on you and your baby. Under certain circumstances, medical interventions are necessary and may even be helpful. However, knowledge of both the natural and assisted birth processes, as found within the pages of this book, will assist you in evaluating the merits of each medical intervention and allow you to consult in an informed manner with the health team you assemble.

In this pregnancy and childbirth guide you will find information on preventing premature birth; natural remedies for common pregnancy problems; the value of hiring professional labor support; and watching and waiting as an alternative to forcing labor. You will read about new, effective pain relief during labor; tips on assisting your baby to descend and rotate more easily; midwife techniques for moving stalled labor; how to create a gentle, safe labor and delivery for your baby; as well as other new and important research that will assist you in making informed, intelligent decisions regarding the heath of your new family.

A Childbirth Resource Directory has been included in this book to help guide you to the best prenatal and postnatal services in your city. Researchers from around the world have contributed vital information that you need to know before you have your baby. Mothers of every age have contributed their practical knowledge and experience on pregnancy, childbirth, breastfeeding and newborn care.

Birth is a normal, natural, empowering experience. Studies show that more than ninety-five per cent of women are capable of giving birth without any medical interference. Women around the world are reclaiming this powerful experience by choosing a safe and gentle birth for themselves and their babies.

Whatever setting you are most comfortable giving birth in; hospital, birthing center or a quiet birth at home, plan on hiring professional labor support for the best result for your entire family.

This book is intended to help you through your childbirth experience while giving you the emotional, physical, spiritual and intellectual support that was once common among a community of family and friends. May this book guide you and give you the confidence to enjoy every stage of your pregnancy and childbirth, and lead you to a safe and gentle birth for you and your new family.

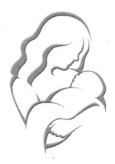

# Chapter One - First Month

Take your home pregnancy test with your partner. Let him share in the excitement or surprise. All pharmacies sell pregnancy tests for less than ten dollars. Pregnancy tests can be used as early as three weeks after the first day of your last period. Spend some time thinking about your conception date and mark this date or dates on your calendar. Your conception date can become very important in the later stages of your pregnancy.

When do you tell people that you are pregnant? Tell your family first! Your family will not want to hear about such an important event from other people and news travels fast. Your friends should be the next to know and then the people that you work with. Be careful at work; your boss may not want to find out from the person at the front desk. Tell all of the other interested parties when you feel comfortable. For some, this is immediately and for others it may be three or four months down the road.

Each day you give your baby in your womb is a precious gift only you can give. Your first baby may easily want to stay in your womb for two or three weeks after an estimated due date of forty weeks, growing and developing safely even throughout the last stages of your labor and delivery when your baby's lungs mature by a hormone released by your contractions during labor. This extra timing is a good thing to keep in mind when scheduling out of town family with your new baby.

Being pregnant isn't like anything you have ever experienced. Get ready to accept that many things will change: the way you feel, the way you look, the way some people talk to you and treat you. You will be changing some of your own ideas as well about parenting once you become a parent. Your sleep habits will change, your eating habits will change to support the growth of your baby, you may experience highs and lows in your energy and emotions. For some women, even their dreams change. Each pregnancy, every woman and every baby is very different from the next. You will also find that each stage of your pregnancy is different from the next, giving you new challenges and joy as your baby grows and takes form within you.

## Calculating Your Due Date

To calculate the estimated arrival of your baby take the first day of your last period and count forward 42 weeks and mark it on your calendar.

Counting fourteen days after the first day of your last period will give you the date of conception if your cycle is usually 28 days long.

Henci Goer, childbirth researcher and author of Obstetric Myths Versus Research Realities, 1995, has reported studies that show the median gestational length exceeds 280 days among healthy, white, middle-class women. Babies of first-time mothers have an average gestational length of 38 to 42 weeks and longer. No person and no machine can give you the exact date your baby will be ready to be born. Sheila Kitzinger, childbirth educator and researcher, reports that seven out of ten babies arrive 10 days after a due date of forty weeks.

## Prenatal Vitamins and Minerals

The day you become aware that you are pregnant; go to a health food store and purchase prenatal vitamins and minerals. Health food stores may offer the best value for the amount invested. If you have planned your pregnancy take the prenatal vitamins and minerals three months before you conceive your baby to help prevent birth defects. Continue to take your prenatal vitamins and minerals throughout each day of your pregnancy and for the first six months after the birth of your baby.

Pregnancy places a high demand on your physical and emotional body and by giving yourself extra nutritional support at this time you and your baby will benefit greatly. Additional nutritional support during pregnancy will also help to prevent birth defects.

## Preventing Birth Defects

The March of Dimes has now found conclusive research that many birth defects can be prevented by taking folic acid (a B vitamin) supplement, especially for the month before you are pregnant and for the first three months of pregnancy. They suggest you consume 0.4 milligrams of folic acid every day. Folic acid is found mainly in green leafy vegetables, beans, asparagus, citrus fruits and juices, whole grain foods and liver. It is difficult to get enough folic acid through diet alone, so it is important to make up the difference by taking a prenatal vitamin supplement. Zinc is also an important mineral that can prevent birth defects.

Research from Nobel Peace Prize Nominee Dr. Joel Wallich, BS, DVM, ND, shows that pregnant women from around the world who naturally consume extra minerals during pregnancy have fewer or no birth defects.

# Natural Remedies for Morning Sickness

Do soda crackers really work? Yes! Leave a package on your bedside table and eat a few before you get up in the morning. Keep some small packages of crackers in your purse in case nausea strikes while you are away from the house.

- Chew on licorice-tasting fennel seeds to calm queasiness.
- Fresh grated ginger and fennel seeds make a comforting tea to settle your stomach. Ginger can be purchased at your grocery store in the fresh vegetable section.
- Try eating your favorite foods from childhood, like ginger ale, jello or whatever your mother fed you when you weren't feeling well.
- Always get up slowly in the morning and take small breaks throughout the day with your feet elevated.
- Hot teas may help, especially spearmint or peppermint, known to be good for indigestion, or try the excellent "women's tea" known as red raspberry-leaf tea. If cold is more appealing, make popsicles or ice chips with the teas.
- Take short walks in the fresh air whenever possible.
- Drink bottled or purified water to flush your system.
- If you feel as though your stomach is not digesting food well, increase your consumption of raw, enzyme-rich foods. Fresh cantaloupe, papaya and pineapple have the highest naturally occurring enzymes of all foods and help a great deal with digestion.
- Make sure you are napping at least once a day to allow your body to recharge. Even a short nap can help you to feel stronger.
- Some health professionals are recommending one tablet of Vitamin B6, in the amount of 50 mg to 100 mg before bed, and this has worked extremely well for some women. Single B vitamins should be used only for short periods of time. Switch to a B-complex vitamin after a two-week period.
- There is a strong connection between nausea during pregnancy and low blood-sugar levels. Make sure you are eating small meals throughout the

day to keep your blood-sugar level up throughout the day and evening.

- A high protein snack before bed can help to alleviate some symptoms.
- Try powdered ginger root in capsules, three capsules a day.
- Slippery elm is a soothing and strengthening herb for the stomach. It has as much nutrition as oatmeal and is so gentle that it can be retained by the most sensitive stomach. It can be taken in powdered form in capsules or made into gruel.
- Carry raisins, raw almonds, rice cakes or whole-wheat crackers with you so that you can keep your blood-sugar level up.
- Blue green algae, such as spirulina, is very high in protein and very easy to digest. Spirulina powder can be mixed with mashed bananas or other fruit and provides excellent nutritional support. It can be taken in tablet form as well.
- Try increasing your water intake to six glasses a day.
- Many women find sea-bands useful. These are elastic bracelets with a plastic button that are worn on the wrist to put compression on an acupressure point that controls nausea. These can be worn 24 hours a day.
- Never take any prescription or non-prescription drugs for your nausea. Benedictin, in the past prescribed by some doctors for the nausea of pregnancy has been associated with birth defects such as cleft palate and heart deformities.
- Consult a midwife or homeopath if you find your morning sickness is not alleviated by the above remedies. Reasons for nausea can be many and varied and getting at the cause can give better direction to the remedy.

## Choosing Your Health Team

Create your health team now. The more responsibility you take for your pregnancy and childbirth, the better the results will be. Be an active participant in your prenatal care. Use your health team as a resource; not an authority. One of the reasons there are so many medical interventions in hospitals, which lead to complications, is because women have not been taught to trust in their ability to deliver naturally and without fear. The full responsibility for the health of the mother and the baby is then shifted unfairly to the doctor's and the nurse's shoulders.

Visit the free-standing birthing center in your city and find out what they have to offer you. Free-standing means to stand free from hospital rules and regulations. Many of the free-standing birthing centers offer you unlimited options for your birth, including water births. Some general practitioners are delivering babies again. You may want to use your family doctor along with a doula who will stay with you throughout your entire labor and delivery. You may decide to have a home birth, assisted by a midwife support team during your pregnancy, labor, and delivery and at home with your baby. Midwives will often work on a sliding fee to accommodate mothers of all incomes, which can be an added bonus. In many countries of the world, including Great Britain, midwives are publicly funded so that every woman can have a choice for the birth of her baby.

After researching your options, it will soon become clear which method of childbirth you will be most comfortable with. To create your health team you may want to include all or some of the following:

1. Midwife, General Practitioner, Obstetrician, Osteopath, or Naturopath
2. Labor Support Coach – Midwife, Doula or Professional Labor Support
3. Birth Partner – Your Partner or Female Relative or Friend
4. Childbirth Educator – For Prenatal Classes
5. Breastfeeding Support – Neighborhood La Leche Group or Breastfeeding Clinic
6. Postnatal Care – Midwife or Doula

Your nearest Childbirth Association or Midwives Association can be an excellent resource center for finding out what your city has to offer. Visit your nearest office for a cup of tea and free information on what your area has to offer. The Childbirth Resource Directory in this guidebook will refer you to the many services that are offered to new mothers in the areas of pregnancy, childbirth, breastfeeding and newborn care. By taking advantage of these services you will create an excellent support team in your city or town for yourself and your baby.

When interviewing health team members, book your appointment for a consultation only. Remind the receptionist upon your arrival that you wish to meet with the doctor in his office for a consultation. If you have chosen your family general practitioner to continue caring for you throughout your pregnancy, make sure that they will be attending the birth of your baby as well. Continuity of care is important for all members on your health team.

Follow your intuition and your feelings when choosing your health team. You have a vision of how you wish your labor and delivery to be; if you find it difficult to get agreement on your birth plan, switch to another caregiver. Make sure your health professionals make time to answer all your questions and that you feel confident in their approach. Don't be surprised if you have to change caregivers. A good working relationship is important for both of you. What is most important is that you both have the same ideas about birth.

Take your time at the beginning of your pregnancy to create a health team that you will be completely at ease with. Your vision of your birth is as unique as you are, and you deserve to have support for it. When choosing your health team, follow your intuition, and ask yourself the following questions:

1. Does my doctor or midwife listen to me?
2. Does my doctor or midwife directly answer all of my questions?
3. Do I feel comfortable with my doctor or midwife?
4. Do I feel respected by my doctor or midwife?
5. Do I trust my doctor or midwife?

The most empowering part of pregnancy and childbirth is the role you will play. By creating a health team and place of birth most comfortable for you, you will become more confident and positive about your role ahead.

When you are discussing birth issues with your doctor or midwife, ask under what circumstances would they perform an episiotomy, induction or cesarean. Ask how their rates of intervention compare to other health professionals in your city or town. Ask if they have experience with normal birth and what percentage of women experience normal birth with them. Find out if you will have professional labor support available to you throughout the entire labor or if the physician only attends during the last few moments of delivery. Don't be surprised that you may be left alone for long periods of time if you are having your baby in a hospital. It is critical to plan for professional labor support to be with you at all times if this will be your first baby.

Be prepared by creating a birth plan to go over with your doctor or midwife. A sample birth plan is shown in the next section and can be modified to fit your design. The following sections explain some of the common medical interventions that can put both you and your baby at risk. Bring this book with you to your first consultation with your health team members and talk about these important issues with your team.

# Fertility Help

Are you unhappy with your current method of birth control or are you demoralized by your quest to have a baby? Do you also experience confusing signs and symptoms at various times in your cycle, but are frustrated by a lack of simple explanations? The book, Taking Charge of Your Fertility, is an invaluable resource that will help you find the answer to your questions while giving you amazing insights into your own body.

Taking Charge of Your Fertility has helped hundreds of thousands of women achieve pregnancy, avoid pregnancy naturally, or simply gain better control of their health and lives. Taking Charge of Your Fertility thoroughly explains the empowering Fertility Awareness Method, (FAM), which in only a couple of minutes a day allows you to: enjoy highly effective and scientifically proven birth control without chemicals or devices, maximize your chances of conception before you see a doctor, or expedite your fertility treatment by quickly identifying impediments to pregnancy achievement, increase the likelihood of choosing the gender of your baby, and to gain control of your sexual and gynecological health. This expanded new edition includes: a revolutionary new, fully intuitive charting system, numerous new master charts, including separate ones for birth control, pregnancy achievement, and menopause, the latest on fertility conditions and high-tech treatments, and comprehensive tables that clearly summarize fertility-related drugs and procedures.

Toni Weschler, MPH, is a nationally respected women's health educator and speaker with a master's degree in Public Health. She founded Fertility Awareness Counseling and Training Seminars (FACTS) in 1986, and has lectured at hospitals, clinics, and universities since 1982. She recently helped develop cycle-tracking software as an adjunct to her book, Taking Charge of Your Fertility. The Ovusoft Fertility Software is available at www.ovusoft.com. She is a frequent guest on television, radio, and Web sites, where she continues to advocate the dissemination of Fertility Awareness education as an empowering body of knowledge for all women of reproductive age.

## Missed Pregnancy/Repeated Miscarriage:

A tremendous amount of guilt, shame and blame can be felt by a mother and father with fertility challenges. Regardless of the reasons for these health challenges, whether the challenges are physical, environmental or a medical mystery, the parents must realize there is no need to feel fault or blame. There are many options available today for fertility challenges. The best thing to do is to create a plan for fertility. Read the section in this book on "How to Prevent Premature Birth" for more ideas on improving the viability of your pregnancy.

# What You Need To Know Before You Have Your Baby: Repeated Miscarriage

"Miscarriage is hard to deal with. It occurs in 15-20% of all pregnancies, usually in the first three months. However, some families will experience multiple miscarriages. After three or more miscarriages, it's referred to as repeated miscarriage or habitual abortion.

Once you've suffered from multiple miscarriages, though the exact number will be determined with the help of your care provider, you might be offered special tests to try and help determine the cause of your losses.

## Causes of Repeated Miscarriage

**Chromosomal:** This is one of the most common causes of miscarriage, comprising over half. It may be a case of problems with the number of chromosomes, the structure of the chromosome, or even the genetic material that they carry. Random, chance problems are the usual cause of genetic problems, however there are times when some genes are repeatedly passed on which can contribute to multiple pregnancy losses.

You and your partner should be tested by a genetics specialist if you are repeatedly passing on chromosomal problems.

**Uterine Anomalies:** Abnormalities of the uterus can be something that you're born with, like a double uterus, a uterus that is divided by a wall (septate), etc. There are also problems with fibroids for some women. These are growths that can occur any place in the uterus, which may have no effect on conception or pregnancy or can cause problems. The good news is that the majority of these problems can be dealt with prior to conception through surgery, thus increasing your chances of a health pregnancy.

**Hormone Imbalance:** Hormonal imbalance can be a problem for some women, usually known as a luteal phase defect, where there is not enough progesterone to sustain a pregnancy. Treatment is usually given in the form of hormones prior to the luteal phase to increase the progesterone or in the form of progesterone supplementation.

Progesterone therapy has been wildly popular and many women and practitioners swear by this form of treatment. However, there are also those who have not found it to be beneficial. The studies available are really inclusive. A look at the potential risks and benefits is advisable for those considering this therapy.

**Immunization Problems:** Sometimes your body will see the baby as a foreign body and attack it rather than accept it. When this happens the mother's body rejects the baby and a miscarriage ensues. There are certain blood tests, which can help determine if this is your problem and there may be medications to help you maintain a pregnancy. It can also be caused by an immune difference between the mother and father.

**Maternal Illness:** Generally a healthy mother, even with a history of chronic illness can have a successful pregnancy. Usually the key to this pregnancy will be diagnosis and control of the underlying factors. Some will have no effect on the pregnancy, while others require monitoring. Here is a list of some of the potential problems:

- Diabetes
- Heart Disease
- Kidney Disease
- High Blood Pressure
- Thyroid Disease
- Infections
- Environmental Factors

Exposure to certain chemicals, drugs, x-rays, etc. have the potential to cause repeated miscarriage. Some of these factors are work related, while others may be related to your life style. Factors like drinking, smoking (first and second hand) do have an impact on pregnancy, for both partners.

## Diagnosis & Future Pregnancy

This can be the difficult part of the process. Sometimes no answer is ever found. However, the process is quite involved. In addition to complete medical history for both you and your partner, you will have a complete physical exam as well. Your exam may include:

- Blood work (hormones, antibodies, disease)
- Genetic Counseling and potential testing (You and your partner)
- Testing for infection in the reproductive organs
- Ultrasound to look for structural problems of the uterus
- Biopsy of the uterine lining
- X-rays of the reproductive tract (hysterosalpingogram)
- Hysteroscopy (Minor surgery to visualize the reproductive organs through the vagina)
- Laparoscopy (Minor surgery to visualize the reproductive organs through the abdomen)
- Testing of any genetic material from previous miscarriages, if available

When to get tested will depend on your feelings and those of the practitioner you are using. Generally having one miscarriage is not a reason to run for testing unless something out of the ordinary is expected. However, it is hard to realize that sometimes there is nothing we can do to prevent the loss of a pregnancy.

### Future Pregnancy

The good news is that even after more than one miscarriage your chance of having a healthy pregnancy is still good. With testing and possible treatment you and your practitioner can hopefully bring down the risks of a future loss. What type of treatment will be necessary will depend on the cause or causes determined. Make sure you talk to your practitioner about what a future pregnancy will be like, what type of special tests or monitoring you might require."

Reprinted with kind permission from Robin Elise Weiss, BA, LCCE, ICCE-CPE, Copyright 2006, All Rights Reserved. Robin Elise Weiss is a mother of seven, a certified childbirth educator, doula and she has attended over 500 births. Her web site, The Pregnancy Birth site at About.com has grown to be one of the largest and most well-read pregnancy sites on the Internet. Her latest book, The About.com Guide to Having A Baby is now available at www.pregnancy.about.com and www.robineliseweiss.com.

(Editor's Note: To locate the references upon which all reprinted articles are based, please refer to the website listed after each author's article.)

## What You Need To Know Before You Have Your Baby: A Look At Today's Fertility Options

"The day Tracy Hammer brought her new baby girl home from the hospital, after battling infertility for nine years, the phone rang. It was me, requesting an interview about her experiences with infertility.

To Tracy Hammer, leader of an Infertility Awareness Association (IAAC), the irony of that chance phone call couldn't have been more poignant. On a day that marked the end of a long and painful road, she sounded wrung out and beaten down from battling against her own body's ill will. And now, just as she was shifting her focus to living her dream, it was time to talk about the muck that had engulfed her and her husband: Nine years of trying, then questioning why her body was betraying her desire to do something as seemingly simple as bearing a child. And then the testing, the surgeries, and the hope, kindled and faded and finally replaced with desperation and despair.

Infertility is described as a medical condition or disease by a myriad of infertility organizations and medical professionals around the world. For a woman who longs to bear a child so much that her breasts ache, it can feel like wearing a barren badge of shame. For men, infertility figuratively and emotionally kicks them in the nuts, causing more breath-stealing pain than any school-yard bully could ever inflict.

Infertility is also a label that some grab on to a little too readily, when that little line fails to appear on the stick after yet another month of trying. In our solution-oriented world, it can be comforting to have a name for not getting pregnant rather than it just isn't happening. Action-oriented couples can then do something about the thickening void that quickly becomes the centre of their formerly carefree existence.

This year marked the birth of the 5,000th baby conceived through in vitro fertilization (IVF) in Calgary, Alberta, Canada. A press conference was held last August; a picnic was organized, and sets of triplets, twins and singletons of all ages showed up for "Generations Celebration 5000" with parents and press all 'round.

The Regional Fertility Program (RFP) is the largest IVF clinic in Canada. According to it's medical director, Dr. C. A. Greene, it boasts one of the highest success rate of live births in the nation – 50 percent (compared to the national average of about 24 percent, according to the Canadian Fertility and Andrology Society). Open seven days a week, it is the only clinic of it's kind in Calgary. Sixty to seventy-five patients file through it's doors daily from the city and out of province, usually after waiting for several months to get in.

The clinic offers the full range of fertility services for both men and women, including treatments such as "super-ovulation", "therapeutic donor insemination", "intrauterine insemination", and other treatments and drug therapies with multi-syllabic names that boggle the mind.

In vitro fertilization is considered by the medical community to be the most effective infertility treatment available today. According to Greene, one "fresh" IVF cycle (using non-frozen embryos) runs about $4,650 CDN plus upwards of $3,000 CDN for drugs needed to push the ovaries into high gear. Every patient and professional interviewed in this story cited an average cost of about $10,000 for just one try at pregnancy using IVF. Subsequent cycles using frozen embryos are a bargain at about $650, not including the drugs.

Many couples who can't afford IVF, or who have male-factor infertility, opt for ovarian stimulation with injectable hormones (Gonadotropins), often followed by intrauterine insemination (IUI). It's less costly than IVF, but also considered less effective.

Dr. Greene says that IVF is usually the last step for couples. A woman may start with a course of fertility drugs such as clomiphene citrate (Clomid), usually taken for about four cycles or months. Technically, any doctor can prescribe a course of Clomid to a woman concerned about her fertility. Many have, especially while waiting to get into the fertility clinic. This is often the precarious first step couples take when entering the infertility roller-coaster.

Hammer has careened around the roller-coaster so many times it's hard to decipher her emotional, physical, psychological journey. She started by taking Clomid, prescribed by a doctor outside of the RFP, but only ovulated a few times, in spite of taking it for "too long" according to Hammer. She also had surgery for polycystic ovarian syndrome (PCOS), which can affect fertility. No go. Still nothing after six years of intermittent drug treatments and other therapies at the RFP. Finally scraping together the $10,000 required for just one IVF course this past year, she became pregnant.

Susan Robinson has been trying to conceive for almost eight years. Also diagnosed with PCOS, she's had drug therapy for that condition, has taken Clomid, undergone IUI and finally opted for IVF two years ago. After three negative cycles, she and her husband decided to take a much needed break and have recently gathered the courage to hit the fertility trail again, as they still have frozen embryos waiting for them at the clinic.

In addition to surgeries and drug treatments, there are also a number of alternative practitioners in the city offering fertility treatments. Dr. Lindsay Dalziel of Healing Touch Health Centre has been treating fertility patients successfully with chiropractic medicine. "Chiropractic is effective if there is nerve interference, because the nervous system needs to go to those reproductive organs." She explains. "Full spine adjustments have also been shown to help with fertility issues.

It's often after being physically, emotionally and financially spent from years of medical interventions and procedures, that patients see an acupuncturist like Leslie Ring-Adams for the first time. Ring-Adams specialized in fertility acupuncture, and is currently conducting a self-funded study with the RFP on using acupuncture in conjunction with IVF.

"Ideally, I'd love to see them before they had to go through all that. About half my patients are going through IVF and for a lot of those people, IVF is not the end of the road. But I talk about fertility, not infertility," says Ring-Adams.

That's the same approach that Dr. Andrea Beaubrun, a naturopathic doctor, uses in the practice that she shares with her husband Arnel, Integra Naturopaths.

"If you're experiencing infertility, medical doctors would start to treat that. I don't start there. We go from head to toe and look at everything from the digestive system to environmental impacts. We really emphasize that both partners come in," Beaubrun adds. And while many doctors rush their patients, she or her husband spend approximately two hours during the initial consultation with a patient.

The foundation of maximizing fertility, according to Beaubrun is nutrition and optimizing nutritional impact to support the functioning of the endocrine system. She also works closely with her female clients to monitor their cycles and uses acupuncture to further balance women's bodies.

Beaubrun is not fond of the term "unexplained infertility" the ambiguous label given to some of her patients. "There has to be an underlying reason," she says. "That's not to say every woman I treat is going to get pregnant. Natural fertility has no guarantees either."Nor does she treat two patients with the same combination of remedies and diet recommendations.

Jennifer Goral was diagnosed with "unexplained infertility" by the RFP, after going through "very thorough" testing, drug treatment with Clomid, three surgeries and three years of "all-encompassing" focus on getting pregnant.

"We were very discouraged, because no one could tell us anything. We didn't have any answers. And we weren't in the financial position to try IVF. We were considering IUI, but spiritually, we were also thinking that God felt that this just wasn't for us and were learning to accept that."Goral finally saw Dr. Arnel Beaubrun, who prescribed acupuncture, put her on a cleansing diet and supplements and worked with her to track her cycles, while working with her chiropractor, and "boom, four months later I was pregnant." After a great pregnancy, her baby girl was born this past July.

About half of the Beaubrun's patients are also going the "conventional route" and they work with them to increase their chances of conceiving through assisted reproductive technology (ART).

Mike Douglas, an acupuncturist at the Ishiyama Shiatsu Clinic was been practicing acupuncture for fifteen years, with upwards of fifteen percent of his patients being fertility cases. He claims, "In the absence of mechanical problems," an eighty percent success rate.

"By the time many of my patients see me, they've exhausted all other possibilities. They've been on drugs, through IVF, surgeries, you name it. They often come to me out of desperation – I've heard it all," says Douglas.

Citing poor diet and high stress as the leading causes of infertility, his acupuncture and supplement treatments set out to correct these conditions. He also expects a woman to be fully engaged in taking care of her body in order to assist in conception. "In other countries people are taught how to take care of their bodies. But here we don't even follow basic nutrition. I think most of this infertility is caused by stress and poor nutrition," says Douglas.

Beverly Hanck, executive director of the Infertility Awareness Association of Canada, (IAAC) in Montreal concurs, adding that she thinks environment also has a huge impact on fertility. She says male infertility is surpassing female infertility due to environmental factors such as working with chemicals and paints from construction sites and from smoking." I've seen guys quit smoking and their wives are pregnant three months later," she says.

Still, she's supportive of all methods of gaining a wee one, whether it's through natural methods, adoption or assisted reproductive technology. "The problem is, the whole industry is set up like a two-tier system. Only those who can afford it get a chance to have a child."

But procreating is about so much more than dollars and percentages. It's about life and well no life. Hence the hot debate. One thing that rankles those who are being knocked sideways by infertility are those insensitive sods who urge them to "just relax" or imply that they just weren't meant to have a baby. "If you haven't been there; you just don't get it." chorus many infertility patients.

It's true, and only those who have withstood the unrelenting ache for a child can understand the prickly pain, as I have. The dreaded infertility label was lapping at my 40 year old world weary heels through two years of miscarriages and non-conception. The gnawing torture truly became the centre of my universe.

So, is giving birth to a baby conceived after years of heartache and drugs and medical procedures a cure for infertility? Or just a solution?

For Tracey Hammer and her husband, at least, that question became moot when they brought a little bundle home from the hospital that hot August day. Seemingly living in a world of ironies, the IVF pregnancy she achieved this past spring, after nine years of trying, ended in miscarriage.

Just a few weeks later, they got a call from the adoption agency they had registered with four years earlier, saying that a couple wanted to meet them for possible placement of their child. One month later, while still recovering from the miscarriage, Tracey Hammer and her husband brought home their newborn and their nine year quest was over. No wonder her voice was quavering when she picked up the phone that day."

Reprinted with kind permission from Avenue Magazine and Susan Pederson. Copyright 2006. All Rights Reserved. Susan is an investigative reporter and mother of two.

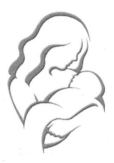

# Chapter Two - Second Month

"Childbirth is a major milestone in a woman's life. It can be a pivotal, positive and empowering experience for a woman." states Dr. Carolyn DeMarco. By taking charge of your pregnancy and the birth of your baby you will enjoy the journey as well as the destination.

Now is the time to read as much as you can, talk to professionals and mothers about birth and work on creating your birth plan and health team for a safe and gentle birth for you and your baby.

## Your Prenatal Visits

Be informed and get information from your health team at every checkup. Throughout the month, write out a list of questions and keep them in your purse; this will save you from "I forgot to ask about...." Ask your questions when you are being examined. No question is too trivial for your peace of mind. Your prenatal check-ups will usually include blood-pressure checks, urine checks and weight checks. When you have many questions, ask the receptionist to book in extra time for you.

Stay in control throughout the entire process. Learn to listen to your body. Inform yourself, read, talk and don't be shy about the physical details. You can lead your health team by being adamant or firm about what you want to take place. Don't settle for less than comfort with your health care team. Trust your feelings about what you want. Being pregnant and birthing your baby doesn't happen every day. If your intuition or instincts are telling you that something is wrong, follow up on that by talking to someone on your team.

One emotion most mothers face is fear. Another one is worry. Deal with both of these emotions as they come up. By asking questions you will eliminate most of your fear and worry. A quick phone call or visit allows most matters to be easily resolved, and your peace of mind during this time is worth it. Bring your Birth Plan along with you at every visit. If you run out of questions you can refer to your plan and talk about each aspect of it in detail.

## Your Birth Plan

Create your birth plan now. Choreograph your baby's first day. Plan every detail of what will be the most exciting and remembered time of your life. As in life, you are the director, script writer, prop person and star. You choose who you wish to have around you in your production. Discuss with your partner and your health team what you want to happen at your labor and delivery. Communicate your wishes by having them prepared in advance. The more you know and are prepared for in advance, the less stress you deal with when you are doing your work during labor.

Birth Plan of: _____

Thank you for choosing to be a part of our health team. It is our belief that birth is a natural event in the reproductive life of a woman. If a medical problem should arise; we expect both the problem and the risks and benefits of any proposed procedure, as well as any natural alternatives to be discussed with us. We would like time alone to consider our options.

We have educated ourselves through monthly prenatal appointments, taking prenatal classes and reading current medical research on pregnancy and childbirth. We appreciate your assistance in guiding us safely through the birth process and your support for the following preferences:

**NO**
Inductions to force or speed up labor.
Intravenous Drugs
Epidural or Spinal Block.
Catheters.
Continual Mechanical Fetal Monitoring.
Ultrasound.
Episiotomy.
Breaking of waters or stripping of membranes.
Unnecessary vaginal exams.
Time limit on labor or delivery.

**YES**

Midwife or Doula present at labor and delivery.

Walking and changing position as much as possible.

Baby monitored manually.

Squatting bar on the birthing bed for delivery.

Shower and bath tub available.

Mirror available for the final stage of delivery.

Sex of baby discovered naturally.

Baby placed upon mother immediately after birth.

Breastfeed baby within moments of birth.

Umbilical cord left intact as long as it continues to pulse.

Partner to cut the umbilical cord.

Baby to be in the room with mother at all times.

Should a cesarean section become necessary partner and professional labor assistant to attend.

Local rather than a general anesthetic if a cesarean is necessary.

Mother would like to welcome baby gently with dim lights, a warm room, baby placed immediately upon mother's breast, warm blankets to be placed over baby and time given for mother and baby to relax and bond.

To labor and give birth in the same place.

To eat and drink as desired.

To have minimum interference.

To be in quiet, peaceful surroundings.

To maintain a spiritual perspective throughout the birth.

To have other children present.

To have other supportive people present.

Signatures of Parents: _____

Nancy Wainer Cohen and Lois Estner state, "Occasionally, once in a while, infrequently, not routinely, each medical or obstetrical procedure can have a place at some birth. For the most part, however, it is best to depend on trusted, knowledgeable individuals rather than technology at birth.

What is needed is a human ear to check the fetal heart, human hands and minds to assess health, in conjunction with feelings and sensory judgment reported by each mother. Birth is a state of wellness. When normal, healthy women say no to the purveyors of technology, they say a confident and loving yes to themselves and their babies."

One physician remarks, "Everyone has their favorite interventions. Dr. A. insists upon IVs but could care less about monitors. Dr. B. demands the use of monitors, but has a nonchalant attitude about IVs. Perhaps the dissension within the field will ultimately provide women with the fuel they need to refuse all but the most necessary interventions."

## Your Emotional Health

Your baby experiences the wide range of emotions you feel. Find a way now to deal with the negative emotions and stress that accumulate daily. What relaxes you? A warm bath, a walk in the fresh air, reading, sewing, hobbies or crafts or exercise can all help you to release your emotions by relaxing you. Incorporate your favorite de-stressing activity into every day so that you can release stress as it comes up.

## Amniocentesis

An amniocentesis test can be done to determine whether your baby has certain genetic defects. Your health plan may cover the cost of the test if you will deliver your baby after your thirty fifth birthday. The risks to you and your baby from this test include infection, hemorrhage, fetal damage, miscarriage, embolism, premature labor, damage to uterine and placental vessels, puncture of the umbilical cord causing cerebral damage, sudden deaths and unexplained respiratory problems for babies at birth. This test has not proven to be accurate on either positive or negative results. The test may show something as wrong when everything is fine. It can easily miss a problem if one exists.

An amniocentesis test is never mandatory. Make sure both you and your partner are made aware of the risks involved. The procedure will be done only after the ultrasound shows that you are at a later stage of pregnancy. During the procedure you lie on your back with your head slightly elevated to relax the abdominal muscles. Your lower abdomen is cleansed with an antiseptic solution and covered with sterile drapes. A needle is then inserted through the skin and into the uterus. Amniotic fluid is withdrawn into the syringe for laboratory testing. Results take at least six weeks, bringing you well into your second trimester before you are informed of them.

If you arrange for an amniocentesis test you must also schedule two days of rest in bed immediately after the test. Your body will need to repair the needle puncture to your womb and to replace the amniotic fluid. Do not exert yourself, avoid any heavy lifting and do not have sexual intercourse the first

24 hours following your test. If you experience any of the following after the first 48 hours following the test, contact your health team immediately: leaking of fluid from the vagina, abdominal pain, cramping or fever.

The scientific validity of amniocentesis has yet to be proven. The inherent health risks have. Make sure you read all the studies before you choose this test. Many hospitals are now including a short seminar on the risks and side effects of this procedure. Ask your health team about the accuracy level of this test before you undertake it and have them explain the rate of error as well. The best way to make certain your baby is healthy is to eat well and rest well. Your health is of the utmost importance to the health of your baby. Taking the best care of yourself and your baby now can give you the best assurance of good health.

## Chorionic Villus Sampling – The New Amniocentesis

Newsweek Magazine in 1992 reported that two separate studies have established a link between the use of Chorionic villus sampling (CVS) and birth defects. The Oxford study and the Humana-Michael Reese Hospital in Chicago both found limb abnormalities in babies who had CVS in utero. The affected children in these studies were born with missing or shortened fingers and toes.

Chorionic villus sampling, which was introduced to the United States in the mid-1980s, consists of removing a small piece of tissue from the Chorionic villi, the hair like projections on the outermost layer of the amniotic sac. Fetal cells present in this tissue are then analyzed and screened for genetic anomalies. Several hospitals have ceased to perform CVS and the National Institute of Health will soon recommend that all women be informed of the risks before agreeing to this procedure.

The Birth Gazette reports that when an expensive test which is undergone to assure parents that their children are free of genetic abnormalities leaves these same children disfigured and handicapped, it is time to seriously consider the absurdity of routine technological intervention.

## Midwives

Midwives are primary caregivers, meaning they care for pregnant women on their own responsibility like a general physician or obstetrician. There are many excellent reasons to have a midwife in attendance throughout your pregnancy, labor and delivery and in your first days at home with your new baby. The ideal choice for assistance with the birth of your baby may be a midwife. A midwife promotes low-tech, woman-centered and family-centered approaches to childbirth. Midwives have experienced the process of birth from both sides and have great empathy with the journey you have undertaken. You can count on your midwife to help you understand the birth process from a woman's point of view.

A midwife will become your advocate and coach during your labor and delivery, with yourself, your partner and your health team. A midwife can enable you to have a better birth by giving you the wealth of experience she has accumulated through her own personal experience and through the experience of hundreds of normal, natural births she has assisted. A midwife will provide the nurturing all mothers need throughout their pregnancy. Midwives work in teams so that you do not have to delay or speed up your delivery at the convenience of your health specialist. You will have one midwife to care for you and one midwife to care for your baby. Midwives are prepared to handle almost every emergency and can arrange transport and attend to you in the hospital should it become necessary. A midwife will help you to create the calm, loving, supportive environment that all mothers want their babies to have.

A nurse-midwife, working in conjunction with obstetricians in a hospital setting does not have the same authority as an independent midwife or a midwife associated with a free-standing birth clinic.

To locate a midwife with a good reputation contact your midwives association or your local childbirth association located in the Childbirth Resource Directory. Go to your library and look for books and articles on midwives, talk to friends and relatives for referrals. When you find your midwife, ask for referrals and call to find out how those births went.

Many women are now choosing to have their second baby in the privacy of their own home, having labor support come in to assist during the later stages of labor. If you feel that your home will provide a better environment for you and your baby or that you may not have your birth plan complied with in your city's hospital, take the time now to read everything you can about home birth or birth in a free-standing birth clinic and find out why many women are now choosing this option. Whether you plan to have your baby at a hospital, a free-standing birth clinic or at home, a midwife can guide you to a safe and gentle birth for you and your baby.

## Doulas

A doula provides emotional and physical support during pregnancy, labor, birth and postpartum. Doulas are called childbirth assistants, labor support professionals, birth assistants or birth companions. A doula is hired by you and sometimes provided by the hospital as your professional labor coach. In the best situation, you would use an independent doula you had met and spent time with prior to going into the hospital.

A doula provides explanations of medical procedures, emotional support and advice during pregnancy, and provides exercises and suggestions to make pregnancy more comfortable. She helps with preparation of your birth plan, provides massage and other non-pharmacological pain relief measures, gives positioning suggestions during labor and birth, and provides support for your partner. She will also help you to avoid unnecessary medical interventions, assist you with breastfeeding and begin a written record of the birth, along with other additional services that vary from doula to doula.

In Mothering the Mother: How a Doula Can Help You Have a Shorter, Easier and Healthier Birth by Klaus, Kennell and Klaus, the authors report that, "The presence of a doula:
- Reduces the overall cesarean rate by 50%
- Reduces length of labor by 25%
- Reduces oxytocin (Pitocin) use by 40%
- Reduces pain medication by 30%
- Reduces the need for forceps by 40%
- Reduces requests for epidurals by 60%."

A doula will charge for her services depending upon her personal experience and any extra services required or offered. Some hospitals in larger cities are now including doula services at no extra charge to their patients.

To find a doula with the experience you require, call your local association for Doulas or Midwives in the Childbirth Resource Directory. They will be able to connect you with a doula who matches your birth plan and the personalities and values of both you and your partner.

## Changing the Birth System

It is up to women as tax payers and consumers to ask our health plan organization to provide the services of midwives, doulas and birthing assistants before, during and after birth for women having their birth in a hospital, birth centre or home environment. If your health plan does not cover professional labor support, take the money out of your savings to pay for the extra service. This is an excellent investment for the future health of mother, father, and baby.

Many women are refusing the standard plan that is being offered by the obstetric hospital system and they are creating their own positive planned childbirth. It is only through knowledge of our options that we will be able to make positive changes in the present birthing system. You can support the various associations now forming to help all women have access to safe alternatives in childbirth. Most of these community associations are listed in the internet and they welcome any and all assistance.

## Shopping Tips

Specialty maternity clothing stores have excellent selections of work and casual clothing, evening wear, lingerie and every accessory you will need for your pregnancy. Maternity stores offer women adjustable clothing so that the pants and skirts purchased will fit you comfortably throughout each stage of your pregnancy. The sales clerks are very supportive and knowledgeable. Visiting the store during the early stages of your pregnancy will help you to begin to plan your new wardrobe around your first basic purchases.

Plan your first maternity purchase to include a pair of solid colored pants or skirt. You will be able to use your regular blouses for some time, so invest your money where you will get the most comfort. Do not let any of your clothing bind you about the waist, hips or breast area. Your body is growing and changing to accommodate your new baby, and your baby needs room to grow and will appreciate the extra breathing space too.

Comfortable shoes are important during your pregnancy. As you gain weight, your feet take the pressure. To avoid ending up with pressure points on your toes, invest in a couple of pairs of comfortable shoes as the key to comfort in the early months of your pregnancy.

### What You Need to Know before You Have Your Baby: Nature's Hormonal Blueprint for Labor

"Giving birth in ecstasy: This is our birthright and our body's intent. Mother Nature, in her wisdom, prescribes birthing hormones that take us outside (ec) our usual state (stasis), so that we can be transformed on every level as we enter motherhood.

This exquisite hormonal orchestration unfolds optimally when birth is undisturbed, enhancing safety for both mother and baby. Science is also increasingly discovering what we realize as mothers -- that our way of birth affects us life-long, both mother and baby, and that an ecstatic birth -- a birth that takes us beyond our self -- is the gift of a life-time.

Four of the major hormonal systems are active during labor and birth. These involve oxytocin, the hormone of love; endorphins, hormones of pleasure and transcendence; adrenaline and noradrenaline (epinephrine and norepinephrine), hormones of excitement; and prolactin, the mothering hormone. These systems are common to all mammals and originate deep in our mammalian or middle brain.

For birth to proceed optimally, this part of the brain must take precedence over the neocortex, or rational brain. This shift can be helped by an atmosphere of quiet and privacy with, for example, dim lighting and little conversation, and no expectation of rationality from the laboring woman. Under such conditions a woman will intuitively choose the movements, sounds, breathing, and positions that will birth her baby most easily. This is her genetic and hormonal blueprint.

All of these systems are adversely affected by current birth practices. Hospital environments and routines are not generally conducive to the shift in consciousness that giving birth naturally requires. A woman's hormonal physiology is further disturbed by practices such as induction, the use of painkillers and epidurals, cesarean surgery, and separation of mother and baby after birth.

## Hormones in Birth

### Oxytocin

Perhaps the best-known birth hormone is oxytocin, the hormone of love, which is secreted during sexual activity, male and female orgasm, birth, and breastfeeding. Oxytocin engenders feelings of love and altruism; as Michel Odent says, "Whatever the facet of love we consider, oxytocin is involved."

Oxytocin is made in the hypothalamus, deep in our brains, and stored in the posterior pituitary, the master gland, from where it is released in pulses. It is a crucial hormone in reproduction and mediates what have been called the ejection reflexes: the sperm ejection reflex with male orgasm (and the corresponding sperm introjection reflex with female orgasm); the fetal ejection reflex at birth (a phrase coined by Odent for the powerful contractions at the end of an undisturbed labor, which birth the baby quickly and easily); and, postpartum, the placental ejection reflex and the milk ejection, or let-down reflex, in breastfeeding.

As well as reaching peak levels in each of these situations, oxytocin is secreted in large amounts in pregnancy, when it acts to enhance nutrient absorption, reduce stress, and conserve energy by making us more sleepy. Oxytocin also causes the rhythmic uterine contractions of labor, and levels peak at birth through stimulation of stretch receptors in a woman's lower vagina as the baby descends. The high levels continue after birth, culminating with the birth of the placenta, and then gradually subside.

The baby also has been producing increasing amounts of oxytocin during labor; so, in the minutes after birth, both mother and baby are bathed in an ecstatic cocktail of hormones. At this time ongoing oxytocin production is enhanced by skin-to-skin and eye-to-eye contact and by the baby's first attempts at suckling. Good levels of oxytocin will also protect against postpartum hemorrhage by ensuring good uterine contractions.

In breastfeeding, oxytocin mediates the let-down reflex and is released in pulses as the baby suckles. During the months and years of lactation, oxytocin continues to act to keep the mother relaxed and well nourished. Oxytocin expert and researcher Professor Kerstin Uvnas Moberg calls it "...a very efficient anti-stress system, which prevents a lot of disease later on." In her study, mothers who breastfed for more than seven weeks were calmer, when their babies were six months old, than mothers who did not breastfeed.

Outside its role in reproduction, oxytocin is secreted in other situations of love and altruism, for example, sharing a meal. Researchers have implicated malfunctions of the oxytocin system in conditions such as schizophrenia, autism, cardiovascular disease, and drug dependency, and have suggested that oxytocin may mediate the antidepressant effect of drugs such as Prozac.

## Beta-endorphin

As a naturally occurring opiate, beta-endorphin has properties similar to pethidine (meperidine, Demerol), morphine, and heroin, and has been shown to work on the same receptors of the brain. Like oxytocin, beta-endorphin is secreted from the pituitary gland, and high levels are present during sex, pregnancy, birth, and breastfeeding.

Beta-endorphin is also a stress hormone, released under conditions of duress and pain, when it acts as a painkiller (analgesic) and, like other stress hormones, suppresses the immune system. This effect may be important in preventing a pregnant mother's immune system from acting against her baby, whose genetic material is foreign to hers.

Like the addictive opiates, beta-endorphin induces feelings of pleasure, euphoria, and dependency or, with a partner, mutual dependency. Beta-endorphin levels are high in pregnancy and increase throughout labor, when levels of beta-endorphin and corticotrophin (another stress hormone) reach those found in male endurance athletes during maximal exercise on a treadmill. Such high levels help the laboring woman to transmute pain and enter the altered state of consciousness that characterizes an undisturbed birth.

Beta-endorphin has complex and incompletely understood relationships with other hormonal systems. In labor, high levels will inhibit oxytocin release. It makes sense that when pain or stress levels are very high, contractions will slow, thus "...rationing labor according to both physiological and psychological stress."

Beta-endorphin also facilitates the release of Prolactin during labor; Prolactin prepares the mother's breasts for lactation and is thought to be important in preparing the baby's lungs and heat-regulating systems for life outside the womb.

Beta-endorphin is also important in breastfeeding. Levels peak in the mother at 20 minutes, and beta-endorphin is also present in breast milk, inducing a pleasurable mutual dependency for both mother and baby in their ongoing relationship.

## Fight-or-Flight Hormones

The hormones adrenaline and noradrenaline (epinephrine and norepinephrine) are also known as the fight-or-flight hormones, or, collectively, as catecholamines (CAs). They are secreted from the adrenal gland above the kidney in response to stresses such as fright, anxiety, hunger or cold, as well as excitement, when they activate the sympathetic nervous system for fight or flight.

In the first stage of labor, high CA levels inhibit oxytocin production, therefore slowing or inhibiting labor. CAs also act to reduce blood flow to the uterus and placenta, and therefore to the baby. This makes sense for mammals birthing in the wild, where the presence of danger would activate this fight-or-flight response, inhibiting labor and diverting blood to the major muscle groups so that the mother can flee to safety. In humans, high levels of CAs have been associated with longer labor and adverse fetal heart rate patterns (an indication of stress to the baby).

After an undisturbed labor, however, when the moment of birth is imminent, these hormones act in a different way. There is a sudden increase in CA levels, especially noradrenaline, which activates the fetal ejection reflex. The mother experiences a sudden rush of energy; she will be upright and alert, with a dry mouth and shallow breathing and perhaps the urge to grasp something. She may express fear, anger, or excitement, and the CA rush will cause several very strong contractions, which will birth the baby quickly and easily.

Some birth attendants have made good use of this reflex when a woman is having difficulties in the second stage of labor. For example, one anthropologist working with an indigenous Canadian tribe recorded that when a woman was having difficulty in birth, the young people of the village would gather together to help. They would suddenly and unexpectedly shout out close to her, with the shock triggering her fetal ejection reflex and a quick birth.

After the birth, the mother's CA levels drop steeply. A warm atmosphere is important; a new mother is very sensitive to temperature and if she cools down significantly, the cold stress will keep her CA levels high, inhibiting her natural oxytocin release and therefore increasing her risk of postpartum hemorrhage.

Noradrenaline, as part of the ecstatic cocktail, is also implicated in instinctive mothering behaviour. Mice bred to be deficient in noradrenaline will not care for their young after birth unless noradrenaline is injected back into their system.

For the baby also, birth is an exciting and stressful event, reflected in high CA levels. These assist the baby during birth by protecting against the effects of hypoxia (lack of oxygen) and subsequent acidosis. High CA levels at birth ensure that the baby is wide-eyed and alert at first contact with the mother. The baby's CA levels also drop rapidly after an undisturbed birth, being soothed by contact with the mother.

## Prolactin

Known as the mothering hormone, Prolactin is the major hormone of breast milk synthesis and breastfeeding. Levels of prolactin increase in pregnancy, although milk production is inhibited hormonally until the placenta is delivered. Levels decrease during labor but then rise steeply at the end of labor and peak with birth.

Prolactin is a hormone of submission or surrender--in primate troops, the dominant male has the lowest prolactin level--and produces some degree of anxiety. In the breastfeeding relationship these effects activate the mother's vigilance and help her to put her baby's needs first.

Prolactin has been associated with nurturance from fathers as well as mothers, earning the additional label "The hormone of paternity". New fathers with higher prolactin levels are more responsive to their babies' cries. Animal studies show that prolactin release is also increased by carrying infants.

The baby also produces prolactin in pregnancy, and high levels are found in amniotic fluid, secreted by the baby's membranes as well as the mother's uterine lining. Prolactin is also secreted into breastmilk, at least in the rat. According to one researcher, "... there is evidence that prolactin plays an important role in the development and maturation of the neonatal [newborn] neuroendocrine [brain-hormone] system.

## Undisturbed Birth

Undisturbed birth is exceedingly rare in our culture, which reflects our ignorance of its importance. Two factors that disturb birth in all mammals are firstly being in an unfamiliar place and secondly the presence of an observer. Feelings of safety and privacy thus seem to be fundamental. Yet the entire system of Western obstetrics is devoted to observing pregnant and birthing women, by both people and machines, and when birth isn't going smoothly, obstetricians respond with yet more intense observation. It is indeed amazing that any woman can give birth under such conditions.

Some writers have observed that, for a laboring woman, having a baby has a lot of parallels with making a baby: the same hormones, the same parts of the body, the same sounds, and the same needs for feelings of safety and privacy. How would it be to attempt to make love in the conditions under which we expect women to give birth?

"When I gave birth to my fourth baby, Maia Rose, I arranged a situation where I felt very private, safe and undisturbed, and had my easiest and most ecstatic labor and birth: one-and-a half hours with an unexpectedly breech baby. I believe that this birth proceeded optimally because of this lack of disturbance, and because of my freedom to follow my own instincts."

Undisturbed birth is possible in a variety of settings, but must always involve a feeling of emotional security for the birthing woman. A familiar and supportive companion, such as a midwife or doula, can play an important role in creating and protecting a private space for the laboring woman, especially in a hospital setting.

# Impact of Drugs and Procedures

## Induction and Augmentation

In Australia in 2002, approximately 26 percent of women had an induction of labor, and another 19 percent have an augmentation--stimulation or speeding up of labor-through either artificial rupture of membranes or with synthetic oxytocin (Pitocin, Syntocinon). In the US in 2002, 53 percent of women reported that they had Pitocin administered in labor to strengthen or speed up contractions.

Synthetic oxytocin administered in labor does not act like the body's own oxytocin. First, Pitocin-induced contractions are different from natural contractions, and these differences can have significant effects on the baby. For example, waves can occur almost on top of each other when too high a dose of Pitocin is given, and it also causes the resting tone of the uterus to increase.

Such over-stimulation (hyperstimulation) can deprive the baby from the necessary supplies of blood and oxygen, and so produce abnormal FHR patterns, fetal distress (leading to cesarean section), and even uterine rupture.

Birth activist Doris Haire describes the effects of Pitocin on the baby:

'The situation is analogous to holding an infant under the surface of the water, allowing the infant to come to the surface to gasp for air, but not to breathe.'

These effects may be partly due to the high blood levels of oxytocin that are reached when a woman labors with Pitocin. Theobald calculated that, at average levels used for induction or augmentation/acceleration, a woman's oxytocin levels will be 130 to 570 times higher than she would naturally produce in labor. Direct measurements do not concur, but blood oxytocin levels are difficult to measure. Other researchers have suggested that continuous administration of this drug by IV infusion, which is very different to its natural pulsatile release, may also account for some of these problems.

Second, oxytocin, synthetic or not, cannot cross from the body to the brain through the blood-brain barrier. This means that Pitocin, introduced into the body by injection or drip, does not act as the hormone of love. However, it can interfere with oxytocin's natural effects. For example, we know that women with Pitocin infusions are at higher risk of major bleeding after the birth and that, in this situation, the numbers of oxytocin receptors in the laboring woman's uterus actually decreases, and so her uterus becomes unresponsive to the postpartum oxytocin peak that prevents bleeding. But we do not know the psychological effects of interference with the natural oxytocin that nature prescribes for all mammalian species.

As for the baby, "Many experts believe that through participating in this initiation of his own birth, the fetus may be training himself to secrete his own love hormone." Michel Odent speaks passionately about our society's deficits in our capacity to love self and others, and he traces these problems back to the time around birth, particularly to interference with the oxytocin system.

## Opiate Painkillers

The most commonly used drug in Australian labor wards today is pethidine (meperidine, Demerol). In one state, 38 percent of laboring women in 1998 were given this drug. In the U.S., several opiate-like drugs have been traditionally used in labor, including meperidine nalbuphine (Nubain), butorphanol (Stadol), alphaprodine (Nisentil), hydromorphone (Dilaudid), and fentanyl citrate (Sublimaze).

The use of simple opiates in the labor room has declined in recent years, with many women now opting for epidurals, which may also contain these drugs (see below) As with oxytocin, use of opiate drugs will reduce a woman's own hormone release, which may be helpful if levels are excessive and inhibiting labor. The use of pethidine, however, has been shown to slow labor, more so with higher doses. This is consistent with the known reduction in oxytocin that natural opiates can cause.

Again we must ask: What are the psychological effects for mother and baby of laboring and birthing without peak levels of these hormones of pleasure and co-dependency? Some researchers believe that endorphins are the reward we get for performing reproductive functions such as mating and birthing; that is, the endorphin fix keeps us having sex and having babies. It is interesting to note that most countries that have adopted Western obstetrics, which prizes drugs and interventions in birth above pleasure and empowerment, have experienced steeply declining birth rates in recent years.

Of greater concern is a study that looked at the birth records of 200 opiate addicts born in Stockholm from 1945 to 1966 and compared them with the birth records of their non-addicted siblings. When the mothers had received opiates, barbiturates, and/or nitrous oxide gas during labor, especially in multiple doses, the offspring were more likely to become drug addicted. For example, when a mother received three doses of opiates, her child was 4.7 times more likely to become addicted to opiate drugs in adulthood.

This study was recently replicated with a U.S. population, with very similar results. The authors of the first study suggest an imprinting mechanism, but I wonder whether it may be a matter of ecstasy--if we don't get it at birth, as we expect, we look for it later in life through drugs. Perhaps this also explains the popularity (and the name) of the drug Ecstasy.

Animal studies suggest a further possibility. It seems that drugs administered chronically in late pregnancy can cause effects in brain structure and function (eg chemical and hormonal imbalance) in offspring that may not be obvious until young adulthood. Whether such effects apply to human babies who are exposed for shorter periods around the time of birth is not known; but one researcher warns, "During this prenatal period of neuronal [brain cell] multiplication, migration and interconnection, the brain is most vulnerable to irreversible damage.

## Epidural Drugs

Epidural drugs are administered over several hours via a tube (catheter) into the space around the spinal cord. Such drugs include local anesthetics (all cocaine derivatives, eg. bupivacaine/marcaine), more recently combined with low-dose opiates. Spinal pain relief involves a single dose, usually of opiate drugs, injected through the coverings of the spinal cord, and is short-acting unless given as a combined spinal-epidural (CSE).

Epidural pain relief has major effects on all of the above-mentioned hormones of labor. Epidurals inhibit beta-endorphin release, and therefore also inhibit the shift in consciousness that is part of a normal labor. This may be one reason why epidurals are so acceptable to hospital birth attendants, who may not be experienced or trained in dealing with the irrationality, directness, and physicality of a woman laboring on her own terms.

When an epidural is in place, the oxytocin peak that occurs at birth is also inhibited because the stretch receptors of a birthing woman's lower vagina, which trigger this peak, are numbed. This effect probably persists even when the epidural has worn off and sensation has returned, because the nerve fibers involved are smaller than the sensory nerves and therefore more sensitive to drug effects.

A woman giving birth with an epidural will therefore miss out on the strong final contractions designed to birth her baby quickly and safely. She must then use her own effort, often against gravity, to compensate. This explains the increased length of the second stage of labor and the extra need for forceps when an epidural is used. Use of epidurals also inhibits catecholamine release, which may be advantageous in the first stage of labor; close to the time of birth, however, a reduction in CA levels will, as with oxytocin, inhibit the fetal ejection reflex and prolong the second stage.

Another hormone also appears to be adversely affected by epidurals. Prostaglandin F2 alpha helps to make a laboring woman's uterus contractible, and levels increase when women labor without epidurals. In one study, women with epidurals actually experienced a decrease in PGF2 alpha, and average labor times were increased from 4.7 to 7.8 hours.

Drugs administered by epidural enter the mother's bloodstream immediately and go straight to the baby at equal, and sometimes effectively greater, levels. Some drugs may be preferentially taken up into the baby's brain, and almost all will take longer to be eliminated from the baby's immature system after the cord is cut. For example, the half-life of bupivacaine -- the time it takes to reduce drug levels by 50 percent -- is 2.7 hours in the adult, but around 8 hours in a newborn baby.

Another indication of the effects of epidurals on mother and baby comes from French researchers who gave epidurals to laboring sheep. The ewes failed to display their normal mothering behaviour; this effect was especially marked for the ewes in their first lambing that were given epidurals early in labor. Seven out of eight of these mothers showed no interest in their offspring for at least 30 minutes.

Some studies indicate that this disturbance may apply to humans also. Mothers given epidurals in one study spent less time with their babies in hospital, in inverse proportion to the dose of drugs they received and the length of the second stage of labor. In another study, mothers who had epidurals described their babies as more difficult to care for one month later.

Such subtle shifts in relationship and reciprocity may reflect hormonal dysfunctions and/or drug toxicity and/or the less-than-optimal circumstances that often accompany epidural births--long labours, forceps, and cesareans.

Incredibly, there have been no large studies of the effects of epidurals on breastfeeding, although there is evidence that babies born after epidural have diminished suckling reflexes and capacity consistent with drug-related effects. One study showed that healthy full-term babies exposed to epidurals during labor were less likely to be fully and successfully breastfed on hospital discharge.

## Cesarean Surgery

Cesarean surgery can be a life-saving operation for mothers and babies, but it is often overlooked that it involves major abdominal surgery. Cesarean delivery increases the risk of maternal death by about four times, and can significantly affect the mother and baby's health in subsequent pregnancies. Cesarean rates are currently 27 percent in Australia, and 27.6 percent--the highest level on record--in the U.S.

Obviously there is a shorter or absent labor with cesarean birth, and the peaks of oxytocin, endorphins, catecholamines, and Prolactin are reduced or absent. Furthermore, mothers and babies are usually separated for some hours after birth, so the first breastfeed is usually delayed. Both will also be affected to some extent by the drugs used in the procedure (epidural, spinal, or general anaesthetic) and for post-operative pain relief.

The consequences of such radical departures from our hormonal blueprint are suggested in the work of Australian researchers who interviewed 242 women in late pregnancy and again after birth. The 50 percent of women who had given spontaneous vaginal birth were the most likely to experience a marked improvement in mood and an elevation of self-esteem after delivery. In comparison, the 17 percent who had cesarean surgery were more likely to experience a decline in mood and self-esteem. The remaining women had forceps or vacuum assistance, and their mood and self-esteem were, on average, unaltered.

Another study looked at the breastfeeding hormones Prolactin and oxytocin on day two, comparing women who had given birth vaginally with women who had undergone emergency cesarean surgery. In the cesarean group, Prolactin levels did not rise as expected with breastfeeding, and the oxytocin pulses were reduced or absent. In this study, first suckling had been at 240 minutes average for cesarean babies, and 75 minutes average for babies vaginally born. The authors comment,

"These data indicate that early breastfeeding and physical closeness may be associated not only with more interaction between mother and child, but also with endocrine [hormonal] changes in the mother."

Other research has shown that early and frequent suckling positively influences milk production and the duration of breastfeeding. The authors of the hormonal study above found that duration of breastfeeding was not affected, and conclude, "...other factors...can compensate for deficient hormonal release."

These studies not only indicate important links between birth and breastfeeding, but also show how an optimal birth experience can influence the long-term health of mother and baby. For example, successful breastfeeding confers advantages such as reduced risk of breast cancer and osteoporosis for the mother and reduced risk of diabetes and obesity long-term for the child. And enhanced self-esteem after a natural birth - which can be a life-long effect -- is a solid base from which to begin our mothering.

The connections between events at birth and long-term health certainly deserve more study. But we cannot afford to wait for years for researchers to prove the benefits of an undisturbed birth. Perhaps the best we can do is trust our instincts and vote with our birthing bodies, choosing models of care that increase our chances of undisturbed- and ecstatic- birthing.

## Early Separation

Even in non-interventionist settings, it is uncommon for the baby to remain in the mother's arms for the first one to two hours. And yet nature's blueprint for this time includes a specific and genetically encoded activation of the brain and nervous system for both mother and baby. For example, when the newborn baby is in skin-to-skin contact, at the mother's left breast (which is where new mothers in all cultures instinctively cradle their babies) and in contact with her heart rhythm, according to Joseph Chilton Pearce, "a cascade of supportive confirmative information activates every sense, instinct and intelligence needed for the radical change of environment ... thus intelligent learning begins at birth."

For the mother also, "A major block of dormant intelligences is activated...the mother then knows exactly what to do and can communicate with her baby on an intuitive level." This awakening of maternal capabilities is well known among animal researchers, who link it to the action of pregnancy and birth hormones on the brain of newly delivered mothers. Such intuitive capacities are sorely needed in our human culture, where we rely so heavily on outside advice from books and experts to tell us how to care for our babies.

When these activations do not occur within about 45 minutes of birth, ...cut off from his mother's nurturing and with none of the encoded expectancies met, the newborn's adrenals continue to release steroids in the face of maximum fear and abandonment. The infant screams for a short time and then silence falls.

The damage caused by separation, Pearce writes, is "...massive and past the point of repair." Like Odent, he believes that our current birth practices are psychologically crippling to babies, mothers, and society as a whole and the evidence in his book is compelling.

## Optimizing the Ecstasy

The following suggestions will help a woman to use her hormonal blueprint and so optimize the experience and safety for herself and her baby. Remember that birth is "orgasmic in its essence" so that conditions for birth are ideally as close as possible to conditions for lovemaking.

Take responsibility for your health, healing, and wholeness throughout the child-bearing years.

Choose a model of care that enhances the chance of a natural and undisturbed birth (for example home birth, birth center, one-on-one midwifery care).

Arrange support according to individual needs; trust, a loving relationship, and continuity of care with support people is important.

Consider having an advocate at a hospital birth- a private midwife or doula is ideal.

Ensure an atmosphere where the laboring woman feels safe, unobserved, and free to follow her own instincts

Reduce stimulation of the neocortex (rational mind) by keeping lighting and noises soft, and reducing words to a minimum.

Cover the clock and any other technical equipment.

Avoid drugs unless absolutely necessary.

Avoid procedures (including obvious observations) unless absolutely necessary.

Avoid cesarean surgery unless absolutely necessary.

Do not separate mother and baby for any reason, including resuscitation, which can be done with the cord still attached.

Breastfeed and enjoy it!

Giving birth is an act of love, and each birth is unique to the mother and her baby. Yet we also share the same womanly physiology, and the same exquisite orchestration of our birthing hormones. Our capacity for ecstasy in birth is also both unique and universal, a necessary blessing that is hard-wired into our bodies, and yet that requires, especially in these times, that we each trust, honour, and protect the act of giving birth according to our own instincts and needs.

Dutch professor of obstetrics G. Kloosterman offers a succinct summary, which would be well placed on the door of every birth room:

Spontaneous labour in a normal woman is an event marked by a number of processes so complicated and so perfectly attuned to each other that any interference will only detract from the optimal character. The only thing required from the bystanders is that they show respect for this awe-inspiring process by complying with the first rule of medicine--nil nocere [Do no harm]."

Reprinted with kind permission of Sarah J Buckley, MD. Copyright 2005, All Rights Reserved. Dr. Sarah Buckley is a family physician, an internationally published writer on pregnancy, birth, and parenting, and mother of four children who were born at home. This article has been previously published in Mothering Magazine, issue 111, March-April 2002, and in Byron Child, issue 5, March 2003. This version updated March 2005. This material has also been further expanded as "Undisturbed Birth: Mother Nature's Hormonal Blueprint for Safety, Ease and Ecstasy", featured in Sarah's book, Gentle Birth, Gentle Mothering: The Wisdom and Science of Gentle Choices in Pregnancy, Birth and Parenting. For this book, and more research about gentle birth and gentle parenting, see www.sarahjbuckley.com.

## What You Need To Know Before You Have Your Baby - Preventing Premature Birth

"Prematurity, birth before 37 completed weeks' gestation, is one of the greatest public health problems in the United States today. Each year in the United States there are over four million births. More than one out of ten of these births is premature, or about half a million annually. Half of all deaths to children before their first birthday are due to pregnancy-related factors; nine out of ten of these deaths are due to prematurity and its complications.

Premature babies – preemies – are more than merely small. They are developmentally unprepared for life outside the uterus. If they survive, they are more likely to have problems with growth and development, which can result in physical and mental disabilities. For example, children who were born premature are more likely to have respiratory problems during childhood, as well as a higher incidence of learning disabilities and problems with speech, hearing, and vision. The more premature the infant, the greater the risk of physical and developmental problems during its childhood.

Maturity is not the only factor influencing how healthy your baby will be at birth and during infancy: birth weight is also very important. Babies who were "small for gestational age" or "intrauterine growth retarded" have not grown as well as they should have before birth. Many of the same factors cause both prematurity and poor growth before birth. When an infant is both premature and growth-retarded, the risks of death or subsequent disability are greatly increased. Every week prematurity is prevented buys valuable time for your baby to grow and mature, and increases the possibilities that he or she will be healthy and well developed at birth.

Special precautions must be taken for premature babies, including administering oxygen, placing them in heated incubators, feeding them special dietary formulas, muffling extraneous sound and light, and protecting their fragile skin. During recent years, there have been great advances in the care of these infants and improvements in their survival rates, but despite modern technology, there is no substitute for full-term gestation.

Prematurity is a complex, universal problem, with no single cause and no single solution. One of the strongest risk factors is if you have had a prior premature birth. Every woman brings a unique set of factors to each pregnancy. Some risks cannot be changed, such as your genetic background, obstetrical history, and age. Others, such as how much and how often you lift, carry, stand, or make other physical efforts can be changed. Most of the pregnancy books on the market focus on preparing you for a labor event that lasts thirteen hours on average. My focus is on the whole nine months of your pregnancy: a short-term investment for the lifelong health of your child and the outcome of future pregnancies as well.

While no one can guarantee that your pregnancy will not be premature, by taking the best possible care of yourself and reducing whatever risks you can, you will greatly improve your chances of having a healthy, well-grown baby born at term.

Ask your health team to review with you how to recognize uterine contractions and what to do if and when they occur. Uterine contractions may be perceived as heaviness in the abdomen or as pain in the middle to lower back, accompanied by a tightening of the uterus. When you feel this heaviness or pain, you should place your hands on your abdomen, at the top of the uterus, to determine if these sensations are accompanied by a tightening or hardening of the uterus. When you squeeze your biceps to make a muscle in your arm, you can feel the muscle go from elastic to hard. When your uterus contracts, you can feel the tightening the same way.

Braxton-Hicks contractions begin during your last trimester and generally increase with intensity as you progress toward your time of birth. You will feel these contractions for very short time periods and then nothing at all for hours or days. These contractions are normal and are your body's way to condition your uterus for delivery.

After you detect uterine contractions, you should determine what you were doing when they occurred. The activities that cause uterine contractions vary greatly from woman to woman. For example, for one woman it may be standing on the train during her commute home, carrying groceries, or hanging wallpaper. For another woman, it may be standing for long periods while shopping, carrying a child in her arms, or vacuuming. For a third, it may be an argument with a co-worker or a stressful session of bill paying. Regardless of the activity, it is important for you to:

1. Recognize that uterine contractions are occurring.
2. Identify what activities bring on the contractions.
3. Stop that activity and sit down, or preferably lie down on your left side, until the contractions subside.
4. Drink at least a glass or two of water, since dehydration can also cause uterine contractions.
5. Call your health team immediately and report your contractions.

True labor pains are rhythmic, even during early labor, occurring every fifteen to twenty minutes. After a few hours, the pains occur about every five minutes. False labor occurs when the painful contractions diminish in intensity after a few hours, and labor does not progress. If you experience a sudden gush of fluid from your vagina, with or without painful contractions, call your health team immediately. Since premature contractions are very difficult to stop once they've started, the best way to prevent prematurity is to prevent premature contractions. It is important for you to understand the physical basis of the relationship between standing, stress, and other factors and premature contractions as well.

When you get home, take another close look at the things you take for granted: how much you stand, how often you go up and down stairs – and make changes wherever you can. Walk through your house and evaluate how you can become more organized. Take steps to reduce clutter in your home which in turn will reduce the amount of housework (and physical effort) in your daily life.

Make an effort to decrease the amount of stair climbing, lifting, carrying, standing, and driving you do. Place stools around your kitchen so that it is easier to sit when you are on the telephone or preparing a meal. Turn over the vacuuming to someone else. Lower the volume of the TV and stereo, and cut down on your exposure to noise in other ways if you can. If possible, get help from friends and relatives with food shopping, chores, baby-sitting, and carpooling. When you are with your children spend as much time as you can with them on the floor so that you are not doing so much lifting. Do not lie flat on your back at any time during your pregnancy as it impedes circulation to your baby.

Modify your work commute by reducing the amount of standing and driving. Ask someone on the bus, subway or train to get up and give you a place to sit down. When you are on the job, make a conscious effort to sit as often as possible. Cut down on the physical efforts you make – lifting, carrying, and so on. Avoid noise and fatigue as much as you can and try to fit in at least two rest periods during the day. Lie down to rest, preferably on your left side to increase blood flow to your heart. Ask your employer to help you modify your work environment to reduce the number of hours you work, or devise a compromise between working at home and at the office.

Emily, a thirty-five-year-old nurse and mother of two preschoolers, worked twelve-hour shifts every Saturday and Sunday in the emergency room of a large urban hospital during her last pregnancy. The working conditions were noisy and stressful; she rarely got to sit down for more than a few minutes, usually didn't finish a meal, and frequently had to help lift patients who were unconscious or couldn't move themselves. At 32 weeks gestation, Emily went into labor during a particularly stressful shift. She was admitted to the hospital and given medications to try to stop her contractions, but within a few hours she gave birth. Her son weighed four pounds at birth and spent a week in newborn intensive care and another two weeks in the newborn nursery.

Beth, a thirty-seven year old professional baker, was pregnant with her second child. Her first pregnancy was fifteen years ago, when she was in college. Divorced from the father of her first child and remarried, both she and her life were very different this second time around. First, she was older and got much more tired by the end of the day than she remembered feeling with her first pregnancy. Second, her daily work was much more stressful and demanding then when she was in college and her work environment was frequently hot and noisy. To reduce her risks of premature delivery, Beth took several important preventative steps. She cut down the number of hours she worked per day from eight to six; she cut down the number of days she worked from five to four; she changed her work hours to when the kitchens were less busy, to reduce stress and exposure to noise; and she sat instead of standing whenever possible. Beth worked this modified schedule for the last eight weeks, then stayed home for the last two weeks of her pregnancy. At 39 weeks gestation, she gave birth to a healthy 7 pound 6 ounce baby girl.

Lifestyle changes are completely under your control. Stop smoking and drinking. Don't take any drug–not even a vitamin or an aspirin – without checking with your health team. Reduce your caffeine intake to fewer than 300 milligrams per day. Follow medical guidelines regarding recreational exercise. You'll soon be able to get back in shape after the birth; don't push yourself to exercise vigorously now.

Eating right is the single most important thing you can do for your baby. Fasting, or going without food for prolonged periods, has been associated with the onset of labor. When the blood sugar level drops as a result of fasting, the body compensates by releasing free fatty acids from adipose tissue which can stimulate uterine contractions. Fasting also causes a release of the catecholamine stress hormones, which also lead to uterine contractions. It is particularly important, therefore, that during pregnancy you eat frequently, every two to three hours, and include breads, fruits or rice or pasta, all of which contain carbohydrates, at each meal.

Iron-deficiency anemia is associated with a 2.5-fold increased risk of prematurity and nearly a 3-fold increased risk of low birth weight. Many women have low iron stores, caused most often by heavy monthly menstrual periods. Other causes of low iron stores can include dieting, especially when meats are excluded, bleeding ulcers or hemorrhoids, and the frequent use of iron-binding medications, such as antacids. Tea and coffee can also contribute to the development of iron deficiency. Foods rich in easily absorbed iron include meat, fish and poultry.

Water is a substance vital to life, second in importance only to oxygen. Like many people, you may not consider water an important part of your diet, but it certainly is! Water plays an important role in regulating body temperature through the evaporation of moisture from the skin and lungs. The loss of 1 to 2 percent of total body water triggers thirst, the loss of 10 percent constitutes a serious health hazard, and a 20 percent loss can result in death. During your pregnancy you should be drinking at least six to eight glasses of water a day. This amount is important to help prevent kidney infections, as well as to prevent dehydration, another possible cause of premature uterine contractions.

Consuming 0.4 milligrams of folic acid per day from at least one month prior to becoming pregnant through the first three months of pregnancy can reduce many birth defects. Make sure you're getting enough iron and calcium, from foods or supplements, and choosing the best vitamin supplement for your needs. Eat small mini-meals throughout the day and evening as you are continuing to nourish your placenta and your baby every moment of the day. We are what we eat, and that goes for your baby too!

There are many things we do not know about prematurity. Sadly, prematurity cannot be completely prevented. However, identifying and modifying your personal risk factors are the best ways to improve your chances of having a healthy, full-term pregnancy."

Reprinted with kind permission from Dr. Barbara Luke. Excerpted from, Every Pregnant Woman's Guide to Preventing Premature Birth – Reducing the Sixty Proven Risks That Can Lead to Prematurity, Barbara Luke, ScD. MPH, RN, RD. Barbara Luke is an Associate Professor and Chief, Division of Health Services Research at the University of Michigan Medical School, Department of Obstetrics and Gynecology in Ann Arbor, Michigan. Over the past thirty years Dr. Luke has published extensively in the areas of maternal nutrition, multiple births, and employment during pregnancy. She is the author, coauthor, or editor of sixteen books, and more than 50 original research papers and over 100 scientific abstracts. Dr. Luke's research has been funded from both private foundations and federal sources. Her book, When You're Expecting Twins, Triplets, or Quads (HarperCollins, 2nd edition, 2004) won Outstanding Book of the Year from the American Society of Journalists and Authors in 2000. She is the recipient of the 2005 Agnes Higgins Award from the March of Dimes for distinguished lifetime achievement in maternal-fetal nutrition. You can find more information at her website at www.drbarbaraluke.com.

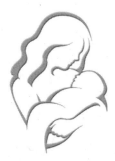

# Chapter Three - Third Month

Above all, enjoy your pregnancy. It's a very special time in your life and it doesn't last long.

Begin now to nap at least once a day. Even thirty minutes a day on your lunch hour will make a difference in your emotional and physical health.

Keep a pregnancy journal if you like. Write your feelings, body changes, thoughts and dreams down. A journal will help you to express yourself and will make interesting reading for your future generation.

Be aware of expectations – yours, your partner, your family and your caregiver. Each person will have a different idea of how the next few months will proceed. Talk over your feelings in detail with each interested party. This may help to dispel any differences in expectations. For example, if you plan to work up to your eighth month, but your partner expects you to work to the end of your pregnancy, you have different expectations. Working out these details before your baby arrives will make your transition to a family smoother.

Plan to eat several small meals a day instead of your usual three. Large meals at breakfast, lunch and dinner do not tend to stay well on your stomach. Eating small meals and having healthy snacks in between is a much better plan. Continue to have mini-meals when your baby arrives and especially when you are breastfeeding.

Keep snacks in your car or desk. Dried apricots or prunes will increase the iron in your blood. Granola bars can give you instant energy and fruit will keep your bowels moving. Your baby and placenta draw nutrition continually from your body, so keep your body well nourished with good foods at all times.

Have a quick snack before you go out if you know you will have to wait a long time before eating.

## Connecting With Your Baby

There is good evidence in support of intrauterine bonding, written and researched by Dr. Thomas Verny in his book, The Secret Life of the Unborn Child. Your love relationship with your baby begins in your womb and expands after birth. Awareness that your baby has an emotional as well as a physical life can help you to feel more connected as you go about your daily activities. Your baby can hear, see, feel and touch while in the womb so that any interaction you choose, like holding your baby in your womb, talking to your baby, playing music to your baby and even just thinking or talking to your baby helps you both to connect at a deeper level.

## Health Danger Signals

If at any time during your pregnancy you feel that either you or your baby are in any danger, go immediately to your doctor or nearest hospital. Do not delay. Always follow your intuition and instincts in regard to your health and your baby's health. Some signals of danger include early contractions, leaking amniotic fluid, any bleeding or spotting, fainting, seeing black spots, cramping or any marked change you may see in your pregnancy that you feel is not normal. Talking to a birth professional at the first sign of a problem will help to turn things around as quickly as possible if there is a problem. Trust your intuition if it is telling you that something is wrong.

## Natural Remedies for High Blood Pressure

High blood pressure is a serious concern to pregnant women. If you have any symptoms of seeing spots before your eyes, swelling of your face, hands or feet, feeling faint or just feeling unwell, have your blood pressure checked immediately. Should you have a problem with your blood pressure, you might want to increase the protein in your diet. Increasing the calcium in your diet can also help. Take the calcium at bedtime with a small amount of food as the biggest drain on calcium stores is when you are sleeping.

If you are experiencing blood pressure problems you must consult a health professional immediately for your sake and your baby's sake. Homeopathic treatments can also assist greatly with this problem. Continue salting your food. New studies are showing salt is critically important during pregnancy. Add either chelated or a liquid calcium supplement to your diet. Organically grown vegetables will also add to your calcium stores, which are being used on a daily basis for your baby.

## Pre-Eclampsia – The Hidden Threat of Pregnancy

Pre-eclampsia, metabolic toxemia of late pregnancy (MTLP) has caused life threatening problems for some mothers. Dr. Thomas H. Brewer has worked with over 7,000 pregnant women providing prenatal care and has found that mothers who eat a protective balanced diet including half a quart of milk, two eggs and two portions of fish or lean meat (with salt to taste) daily can prevent eclampsia. Women following this program did not have a single case of eclampsia, no toxic abruptio placentae and no maternal death. Dr. Brewer also mentions that, so far, United States and Canadian health professionals still insist the cause of eclampsia is unknown.

## Preventing a High-Risk Pregnancy

Dr. Thomas H. Brewer's simple common-sense message to mothers for preventing a high-risk pregnancy is to eat for two, three or four. Avoid all drugs, street and doctor prescribed. Salt to taste, water to thirst, exercise and rest when tired.

Dr. Joel Wallach, BS, DVM, MD, Nobel Prize Nominee, one of the world's leading nutrition experts, has found that over 98% of all animal and human deaths are now caused by nutritional deficiencies. Lack of calcium alone causes over 180 diseases in modern man. Pregnancy draws calcium from all of your stores.

Many common pregnancy problems like intense food cravings, high blood pressure, bleeding gums, muscle cramping, morning sickness, low blood sugar, chronic lower-back pain and other discomforts are caused by a lack of calcium, selenium, chromium, copper, and the fifty other minerals that are just as important, as vitamin supplements during pregnancy. Before you reach for a glass of milk, Tums or calcium tablet, you should know your body will absorb less than 10% from any of these sources. Combining the expertise of these two physicians can help assure you of having a healthy pregnancy and a healthy baby.

## Natural Remedies for Constipation

Being unable to move your bowels on a regular basis can cause your blood pressure to rise dangerously high. Make certain your prenatal vitamins are low in iron to prevent constipation. If you are finding constipation is still a problem, increase the amount of raw fruits and vegetables in your diet.

Excerpted from Take Charge of Your Body, Dr. Carolyn DeMarco, 7th Edition.

"During pregnancy your body produces a hormone called progesterone. This hormone has the effect of relaxing the smooth muscles of your small and large intestines. Thus food passes through your intestines more slowly. Also your growing uterus may press on and displace the intestines. Another major factor contributing to constipation is taking iron supplements.

1. Drink plenty of fluids. Some suggest six to eight glasses of fluid a day. This fluid should consist of pure water, fruit juice or herbal teas.
2. Eat food that is high in fiber such as fresh fruit, vegetables and whole grains. Cut down or eliminate red meat, which is very constipating. Chicken or fish can be eaten instead.
3. One to two tablespoons of unsulphured blackstrap molasses in warm water once or twice a day is a reliable old remedy for constipation. Molasses is also high in iron and trace minerals. Be sure to brush your teeth well after you take molasses.
4. Some women find that drinking eight ounces of prune juice daily keeps their bowels moving.
5. Unrefined bran can be taken daily with whole grain cereal.
6. Ground flax seed, two tablespoons in water twice a day or Metamucil without sugar are two mild laxatives that can be taken safely throughout pregnancy.
7. Discontinue your iron tablets or switch to a less constipating brand or a liquid iron, like Floradix, available in health food stores. I also have had great success with NutriChem iron, which is completely non-constipating.
8. Walk or do some type of physical exercise every day. This promotes regular bowel movements.
9. For some, changing position while sitting may help. For example, the backless chairs, where your knees are lower than your hips.
10. When you are pregnant, the timing of your bowel movement changes. Never sit on the toilet for long periods of time or strain during bowel movements as this can contribute to the development of hemorrhoids. If the stool is not passing easily, force yourself to get off the toilet and go about your business until you really have to go and the stool will then pass more easily."

## Over The Counter Drugs

Stay away from all over-the-counter headache remedies, cold medications, aspirin, or anything that has not been prescribed by your doctor. If you have a persistent cold that is wearing you down, go to your neighborhood health food store or see a homeopathic doctor for a natural remedy.

# Tobacco

Stop smoking. Many birth defects have been linked to the chemicals in tobacco smoke. Cigarette smoking cuts the amount of oxygen available in the maternal blood, which directly affects the growth of fetal tissue. Seek professional help if you are unable to stop smoking on your own.

# Alcohol-Fetal Alcohol Spectrum Disorder

Fetal alcohol spectrum disorder (FASD) describes a spectrum of permanent and often devastating birth defect syndromes caused by maternal consumption of alcohol during pregnancy. The main effect of fetal alcohol exposure is brain damage. This can be caused during any trimester, because the fetus's brain continues to develop throughout the entire pregnancy.

There are a number of subtypes, including standard fetal alcohol syndrome (FAS), and the less noticeable, but sometimes equally serious, possible fetal alcohol effects (PFAE). The latter is also known as prenatal exposure to alcohol (PEA) or alcohol-related neurodevelopmental disorder (ARND).

Features of FASD may include facial deformities, stunted physical and emotional development, memory and attention deficits, a tendency to impulsive behavior, inability to reason from cause to effect, a failure to comprehend the concept of time, difficulty telling fantasy from reality, inability to control sexual impulses, and an apparent lack of remorse.. Secondary disabilities such as mental illness and drug addiction are also likely to develop. Unlike the primary disabilities, these do not reflect the central nervous system damage, but instead develop because the child has difficulty adapting to his environment.

Fetal alcohol exposure is regarded by researchers as the leading known cause of mental retardation in the Western world. In the United States alone, it is estimated that, every year, one in 750 babies born suffers from FAS, and 40,000 from PFAE. The lifetime medical and welfare costs of each child are estimated by some to be as high as US$5 million.

Do not drink alcohol during your pregnancy. Each day another part of your baby is growing or being developed; even one drink can stop or slow down this development. Make a commitment to yourself and your baby to eliminate any consumption of alcohol during your pregnancy.

Fetal Alcohol Syndrome can happen at any stage during your pregnancy if you drink alcohol. Any alcohol you drink is transmitted directly into your womb and concentrates in your baby's brain tissue, perhaps leaving your baby with permanent, irreversible organic brain damage.

View the Fetal Alcohol Syndrome films at your local library to see what challenges these children must face to become aware of the full impact drinking alcohol may have on your baby. If you are unable to stop drinking on your own, seek professional help immediately.

# Nutrition during Pregnancy

"It is important to the health of both mother and fetus that the mother eats a well-balanced and varied diet. Fresh fruits and vegetables, whole grains, legumes, beans, and fish are essential. Limit refined sugars, processed foods, and saturated fats. Organically grown produce, meats, and poultry are preferable. However, if produce is not organic, it should be washed to remove as much of the agricultural chemicals as possible.

Most physicians recommend eating plenty of dairy products during pregnancy, due to their calcium and protein content. Other doctors are more wary about suggesting dairy as a mainstay of a pregnant woman's diet. Lendon Smith, MD, a pediatrician and author of several books on children's nutrition, explains, "Many babies will develop milk sensitivity before they are born because the mother followed the obstetrician dictum: 'Drink a quart of milk every day so the baby will get the calcium.' If a mother is already sensitive to dairy products and takes in milk, cheese, and ice cream, she may not be absorbing the calcium from those foods she is ingesting." Foods such as nuts, soybean products, such as tofu and soy milk, and goat milk products provide alternative sources of protein. Seaweed, green vegetables, and a mixture of sunflower, sesame, and pumpkin seeds are alternatives for calcium. No one food, including dairy, should be eaten on a daily basis, says Dr. Smith, as this practice increases an individual's chance of developing food sensitivities. Contrary to popular belief, a well-chosen vegetarian diet is healthy for a pregnant woman. Vegetarians, who consume no animal products at all, including dairy and eggs, should use a B12 supplement.

Eating five to six small, nutrient-dense meals a day is a sensible idea. Restricting weight gain, which was very popular twenty years ago, was thought to ease a woman's labor. We now know that this is not necessarily so. New guidelines, issued in June 1990 by the Institute of Medicine in Washington, D.C. recommend increased weight gains for healthy pregnant women. The range of optimal weight gains depends on the weight of the mother early in pregnancy: twenty-eight to forty pounds for "underweight women", fifteen to twenty-five pounds for "overweight women", and a maximum of fifteen pounds for "obese women". These new guidelines "reflect current interests in preventing low-birth weight babies and thus reduce the incidence of infant mortality and mental and physical retardation.

Pregnancy is not the time to diet. Dr. Linton offers a simple formula. "If you are eating a whole foods diet, drinking plenty of water, and getting adequate exercise such as walking or swimming, then the weight you gain in your pregnancy is appropriate."

Opinions vary on the amount of protein that is needed during pregnancy. Some experts advocate consuming even more protein than the Recommended Daily Allowance: "I think that dietary protein," says Dr. Birdsall "is probably the most common nutrient deficiency in pregnancy." Pregnant women need seventy to one hundred grams of protein daily, which most people will not get with a normal diet. "These levels of protein," adds Birdsall, "help feed increasing blood volume and guard against complications during pregnancy, such as pre-eclampsia, a potentially dangerous condition characterized by high blood pressure, swelling and/or protein spilling into the urine."

Sodium is needed to maintain fluid balance and blood volume. For this reason, salt restriction is one common nutritional advisement that does not apply during pregnancy. Restricting sodium and using diuretics, once routine treatments to prevent pre-eclampsia and swelling, are not only unnecessary, but potentially harmful. It is best to use salt to taste.

Reprinted with kind permission from Alternative Medicine: The Definitive Guide, by The Burton Goldberg Group, 1995.

# Nutrition

Do not go on any calorie-reduced eating program while you are pregnant. The single most important thing you can do for your baby is to make sure you are eating well and eating often.

Our bodies are primarily composed of water and protein. Include protein with every meal. The most easily digested proteins are eggs, chicken, turkey and white fish.

Your personal need for water may change from day to day. If your urine is clear you can be assured that you have consumed enough water for that day. You will get your best value from the water you drink if you make sure to bring a portable water bottle along with you as you go throughout the day.

A change in the food you purchase can make a vast difference in the health of your baby. If possible, purchase your fruits and vegetables organically. An organic tomato has 2,000 times more iron than a regular tomato. Organic lettuce has 60 times more calcium than regular lettuce.

Reduce the amount of sugar in your eating habits. Chocolate, pop, candy, ice cream and the like will stick to your thighs like gum. Junk food fills you up so that there is no room for good nutritious food.

Ask for water instead of pop with your food. Ask for herbal non-caffeinated tea instead of coffee. Some of the best teas during pregnancy are red raspberry leaf tea, peppermint and ginger.

Wean yourself from regular coffee to half and half and then to decaffeinated coffee.

At parties, bring along a bottle of club soda without sodium, or try some non-alcoholic wine or beer. Or ask for a glass of water with a twist of lime or lemon.

## Single and Pregnant

If you do not have a partner, think responsibly about what is best for you and your baby. You do have choices. Today a mother can have contact with adoptive families throughout the life of their child if that is your choice. A baby gives very little back to a parent initially and demands are on a twenty-four-hour clock. It is a tremendous burden of responsibility to bear alone.

Keep in mind that when you are older you may have a greater wealth of resources to draw upon and remember that a woman's fertility can continue into her forties. You may want to look at adoption if you find yourself without a partner, take the time to discover all your options. Look on the internet under adoption for the agencies operating in your area and interview two or three of the agencies to see if this option is right for you.

On the other hand, some women are raising their children alone in today's society by choice or circumstance. It is a more difficult choice, but possible.

This is an intensely personal choice and one that each woman faces alone. There is no "right" answer or decision in this matter. Don't feel pressured into making a quick decision. Take your time to look at all of your options.

## Your Relationship

The first year with the first baby is considered the most hazardous time for every relationship. In this crucial adjustment year, husbands are more likely to feel insecure about being displaced by the baby, and their wives may feel abandoned, overwhelmed with feelings of inadequacy, fear or discouragement. Be aware that a baby will add more stress to your relationship and make sure that your relationship is strong and that both of you are in agreement on having a baby.

Both partners need an opportunity to vent frustrated and discouraged feelings in an accepting and supportive environment. Make sure you deal with issues as they arise and work together with your partner to find creative solutions to individual problems as they come up. Many couples report a decline in the mutual satisfaction of their relationship after the birth of their first child. Have a plan to increase satisfaction in your relationship. You might want to contact an older couple with children to act as mentors or a marriage counselor to help you work through the rough spots.

# Shopping Tips

Purchase good bras and maternity panties. A great bra for small to medium-size breasts is the sport type with hooks or snaps at front; they are made of Lycra elastic with wide shoulder straps. Sport-type bras keep everything in place and will stretch as you grow. If your breasts are larger make sure the shoulder strap on your bra is at least one inch across, as this will help in the distribution of weight and will stop the strap from cutting into your skin.

Cotton clothes absorb perspiration and are more comfortable than synthetics, especially in the summer months.

Go through your closet and put away all the clothing items you feel will be unsuitable for the months ahead. Plan to shop for maternity wear once a month rather than purchasing your entire wardrobe at once. Your needs will change as you progress along your pregnancy and shopping for a new article each month will give you the lift you need.

## What You Need To Know Before You Have Your Baby: Ultrasound - Weighing the Propaganda Against the Facts

"Women believe that they can ensure the well-being of their babies by having ultrasound scans and that early detection of a problem is beneficial for these babies. That is not necessarily so, and there are a number of studies which show that early detection of some problems with ultrasound might itself be harmful.

In response to women's desire for information about the implications of routine ultrasound examinations, Jean Robinson and I wrote Ultrasound Unsound? in which we reviewed the research evidence and drew attention to some of the hazards (Beech and Robinson, 1996). Since then more evidence has accumulated.

### Miscarriage and perinatal death

It is ironic that women who have had previous miscarriages, or who have conceived after infertility treatment, often have additional ultrasound examinations in order to "reassure" them that their baby is developing properly. Would they consent if they knew of possible increased risks of miscarriage or premature labour or birth?

Obstetricians in Michigan (Lorenz et al, 1990) studied 57 women who were at risk of giving birth prematurely. Half were given a weekly ultrasound examination; the rest simply had pelvic examinations. Preterm labour was more than doubled in the ultrasound group - 52% - compared with 25% in the controls. Although the numbers were small the difference was statistically significant and unlikely to have emerged by chance.

In a large randomized controlled trial from Helsinki (Saari-Kemppainen et al, 1990) which randomly divided over 9,000 women into a group who were scanned at 16-20 weeks, compared with those who were not, there were 20 miscarriages after 16-20 weeks in the screened group and none in the controls.

A later study in London (Davies et al, 1992) randomized 2,475 women to routine Doppler ultrasound examination of the umbilical and uterine arteries at 19-22 weeks and 32 weeks compared with women who received standard care without Doppler ultrasound. There were 16 perinatal deaths of normally formed infants in the Doppler group compared with 4 in the standard care group.

We cannot say whether these studies represent greater risks for everyone, since ultrasound exposure varies so much from one machine to another. It is not, however, only antenatal clinic patients who may be at risk. Physiotherapists use ultrasound to treat a number of conditions. A study done in Helsinki (Taskinen et al, 1990) found that if the physiotherapist was pregnant, handling ultrasound equipment for at least 20 hours a week significantly increased her risk of spontaneous abortion. Also, the risk of spontaneous abortions occurring after the tenth week was significantly increased for deep heat therapies given for more than 5 hours a week and ultrasound more than 10 hours a week.

## Diagnosis of placenta praevia

The Saari-Kemppainen study also revealed the lack of value of early diagnosis of placenta praevia. This is a condition where the placenta is low in the womb and obstructs the opening into the cervix. Of the 4,000 women who were scanned at 16-20 weeks, 250 were diagnosed as having placenta praevia. Because the womb stretches during pregnancy, when it came to delivery there were only four who actually had the condition. Interestingly, in the unscanned group there were also four women found at delivery to have placenta praevia. All the women were given caesarean sections and there was no difference in outcomes between the babies. Indeed, there are no studies which demonstrate that early detection of placenta praevia improves the outcome for either the mother or the baby. The researchers did not investigate the possible effects on the 246 women who presumably spent their pregnancies unnecessarily worrying about having to have a caesarean section and the possibility of a sudden hemorrhage. We now know that stress alone may restrict the baby's growth in the womb.

Since the publication of Ultrasound Unsound?, further studies have raised questions about the value of routine ultrasound scanning.

## Babies with serious defects

The only way in which mass antenatal ultrasound screening has been proved to reduce perinatal mortality statistics is by detection of serious problems at 18-20 weeks and mothers choosing termination. Babies which would have died anyway from lethal conditions die sooner and do not appear in birth statistics. The perinatal mortality rate is reduced but babies lives are not saved.

Almost all babies receive a dose of ultrasound, but even at the best centers, wide variations occur in detection rates for babies with major abnormalities and even in the best centers, antenatal detection rates for heart problems are not high. Both local and international detection rates differ widely in published studies (which are usually undertaken in centers of excellence), but the majority of mothers will be exposed to older machines in ordinary hospitals and clinics. Low detection rates (either from poor equipment or unskilled operators) means all the babies get the ultrasound dose but few of them get the 'benefits' of accurate diagnosis. The skill of the operators will vary (everybody has to learn sometime) but even with the best machines and the best operators misdiagnoses occur. AIMS has had a number of problems with inaccurate diagnosis from portable hand held scanners used on the ward - usually by inexperienced junior doctors.

A study from Oslo (Skari H et al, 1998) looked at how many babies born with serious defects had been diagnosed by antenatal scans, and whether the early diagnosis made any difference to the outcomes. Women in Norway have a scan at 17-21 weeks done by trained midwives, who refer to obstetricians if an abnormality is suspected.

*Knowing about the problem in advance did not benefit these babies; more of them died.* They got delivered sooner, when they were smaller, a choice that could have long-term effects. All 12 babies with abdominal wall defects survived. But for the 6 detected on the scan, their length of hospital stay was longer and they spent longer on ventilators, though the numbers are too small to be significant. They were operated on sooner (4 hours rather than 13 hours) but the short term outcomes were the same. The survival rate in the diagnosed group was 77% and 96% in those who were not detected until after birth.

As well as false negatives (undetected abnormalities) there are also false positives (mistaken diagnosis of abnormalities which don't exist). Such screening carries the risk of termination of a normal pregnancy. Some of these are reported in the literature but we know of other cases.

Although small, this is an important study because pregnant women often automatically assume that antenatal detection of serious problems in the baby means that lives will be saved or illness reduced.

## Growth Retarded Babies

One of the promises held out by antenatal scanning is that obstetricians will be able to identify the baby with problems and do something to help it and great attention is paid to whether the baby is growing normally. A German study from Wiesbaden hospital (Jahn A et al, 1998) found that out of 2,378 pregnancies only 58 of 183 growth retarded babies were diagnosed before birth. Forty-five fetuses were wrongly diagnosed as being growth retarded when they were not. Only 28 of the 72 severely growth-retarded babies were detected before birth despite the mothers having an average of 4.7 scans.

The babies diagnosed as small were much more likely to be delivered by elective caesarean - 44.3% compared with 17.4% for babies who were not small for dates. If the baby actually had intrauterine growth retardation (IUGR) the section rate varied hugely according to whether it was diagnosed before birth (74.1%) or not (30.4%).

So what difference did diagnosis make to the outcome for the baby? Pre-term elective delivery was 5 times more frequent in those whose IUGR was diagnosed before birth than those who were not. 77% of these were the result of medical interventions because of suspected fetal distress and not related to premature labour or rupture of membranes. The average diagnosed pregnancy was 2-3 weeks shorter than the undiagnosed one. The admission rate to intensive care was 3 times higher for the diagnosed babies.

## The Long-Term Emotional Impact

The effects of screening on both parents can be profound. For example, women waiting for the results of tests may try not to love the baby in case they have to part with it. The medical literature has little to say about the human costs of misdiagnosis unless the baby was mistakenly aborted, and even then it tends to focus on legal action. However, a letter in the British Medical Journal revealed how a diagnosis of a minor anomaly can have serious long-term implications for the family:

A woman was referred for amniocentesis during her second pregnancy on the grounds of maternal age (35 years) and anxiety; she was accompanied by her husband. Their normal three year old son played happily during the consultation. The husband confided to the doctor that they had opted for amniocentesis to avoid having another 'brain damaged' child. On questioning it became apparent that an ultrasound examination before their son's birth had shown a choroid plexus cyst. Despite having a healthy child, the husband remained convinced that this cyst had caused his son to be disabled. (Mason G and Baillie C, 1997). This is one of many cases where an abnormal test - even if it turns out to be wrong - can do long term damage to relationships between parent and child (Robinson J, 1997)

As Theresa Marteau, an expert in psychological problems in screening, warned 10 years ago: "Unless the emotional and behavioural consequences of such screening programmes are properly monitored, we will not know their true costs and hence net benefits. We will be uncertain of their value for many and even of whether they should be provided at all" (Marteau T, 1989).

## Evaluating the Risks

When ultrasound was first developed researchers suggested that "the possibility of hazard should be kept under constant review" (Donald I, 1980) and they said that it would never be used in early pregnancy under three months, this initial caution was ignored.  As soon as vaginal probe ultrasound was developed, which could get good pictures in early pregnancies (and get nearer to the baby giving it a bigger dose) it became widely used for dating pregnancy and is claimed to be more accurate. However, a recent article from Denmark (Olsen O and Clausen J, 1997) challenged the widely held view that scan dating of pregnancies is more accurate than counting days from the last menstrual cycle.

The problem is, the authors say, that the time-honored method has always estimated length of pregnancy as 280 days from last period, whereas a study of over 400,000 pregnancies where dates were sure, showed that the actual length was most likely to be 283 days.  So this method often led to an under-estimate. Scanning, on the other hand, was more likely to overestimate pregnancy length by two days. The most accurate assessment would be made by either adding 3 days to the old calculations of time since the last period, or taking 2 days off the estimated scan date. As a result of this study it will no longer be possible to claim that an ultrasound scan is more accurate than using a calendar and the date of your last period.

AIMS has had a number of complaints from women who were certain of their dates but doctors insisted they were wrong because the scan must be right. They believed the technology rather than the woman - sometimes with tragic results.

Research by Liebeskind revealed "the persistence of abnormal behaviour ... in cells exposed to a single dose diagnostic ultrasound ten generations after insonation".  She concluded, "If germ cells were ... involved, the effects might not become apparent until the next generation" (Liebeskind, 1979). When asked what problems should be looked for in human studies, she suggested: "Subtle ones.  I'd look for possible behavioural changes, in reflexes, IQ, attention span (Bolsen B, 1982).

Because ultrasound has been developed rapidly without proper evaluation of its risks and benefits it is now extremely difficult to prove that ultrasound exposure causes subtle effects or indeed any effects, because we simply do not have a sizeable population of pregnant women whose babies did not get ultrasound for comparison. (After all, it took over ten years to prove that the gross abnormalities found in some newborn babies were caused by thalidomide). However, there are a number of ultrasound studies which raise serious questions that still have to be addressed.

The first evidence we saw of possible damage to humans came in 1984 when American obstetricians published a follow-up study of children aged 7 to 12 years born in three different hospitals in Florida and Denver, who had been exposed to ultrasound in the womb (Stark et al, 1984). Compared with a control group of children who had not been exposed they were more likely to have dyslexia and to have been admitted to hospital during their childhood, but no other differences were found. Because this was not a randomized study, it was too easily dismissed. It did not prove there was a problem but gave early warning that there might be.

In 1993 a study in Calgary, Alberta, which examined the antenatal records of 72 children with delayed speech of unknown cause were compared with those of 142 controls who were similar in sex, date of birth and birth order within the family. The children were similar in social class, birth weight and length of pregnancy. The children with speech problems were twice as likely as controls to have been exposed to ultrasound in the womb. 61% of cases, and only 37% of controls, had had at least one exposure. Once again, because it was not a randomized study but was looking back at children after the event its results were not accepted as proved and were dismissed. That does not mean, however, that the results were not valid.

AIMS pressed the Medical Research Council to do a randomized controlled trial without success but the Norwegians, to their credit, did a large scale prospective trial where half the women had two low dose ultrasound scans and half did not.

A Norwegian study (Salvesen K, 1993) showed an increase in left handedness, but no increase in dyslexia. While the increase in left handedness was not large, it was significant and it does suggest that ultrasound may have an effect on the development of the brain. It should be noted, however, that the scanners used in this study emitted very low doses of ultrasound - lower than exposures from many machines nowadays - the women had only two exposures and it was real time, not Doppler, a more powerful form of ultrasound.

## Assessing the Risks

*"Present day ultrasonic diagnostic machines use such small levels of energy that they would appear to be safe, but the possibility must never be lost sight of that there may be safety threshold levels possibly different for different tissues, and that with the development of more powerful and sophisticated apparatus these may yet be transgressed"* (Donald I, 1979).

Donald's foresight was remarkable. The machines in use today are far more powerful than the machines used a decade or more ago, and new variants are being developed all the time. The numbers of routine scans for even a normal low-risk pregnancy are increasing, and the duration of each scan appears to be longer than ten years ago. Yet, there has been inadequate research into the potential long-term effects of these developments.

Measuring the impact of any intervention in pregnancy is very complicated because there are so many things to look at. The child's intelligence, personality, growth, sight, hearing, susceptibility to infection, allergies and subsequent fertility, are but a few factors which, if affected, could have serious long-term implications, quite apart from emotional effects on families when babies have a false positive or false negative diagnosis of some sort of abnormality. Because a baby grows rapidly, exposing it to ultrasound in utero at 8 weeks can have different effects to exposure at for example, 10, 18 or 24 weeks (this is one of the reasons the potential effects of exposure are so difficult to study). Undertaking an ultrasound examination at 8 weeks can have different implications to one undertaken at 24 weeks. Women are now exposed to so many different types of ultrasound: Doppler scans, real-time imaging, triple scans, external fetal heart-rate monitors, hand held fetal monitors. Unlike drugs, whereby every new drug is required to be tested and shown to have benefits that outweigh any possible harmful adverse effects, the rapid development of each new variation of ultrasound machine has not been accompanied by similar careful evaluation by controlled large scale trials prior to being let loose on the unsuspecting public.

Despite decades of ultrasonic investigation, no one can demonstrate whether ultrasound exposure has a particular adverse effect at a particular gestation, whether any ill-effects of ultrasound might be cumulative, or whether they might relate more directly to the output of a particular machine or the length of the examination. How many exposures are too many? What is the mechanism by which fetal growth may be affected? A large randomized study (Newnham et al, 1993) of women exposed to five Doppler examinations during their pregnancies (compared with a control group which had single ultrasound imaging at 18 weeks) showed decreased birth weight, although a later study showed the children caught up later.

There is, in effect, a presumption of safety in the use of this technology (rather as there was for 20-30 years when pregnant women were told that x-rays were absolutely safe, subsequent research revealed an increased rate of cancer in the exposed children). The published studies raise serious concerns which are widely ignored and more and more women and babies are exposed to ultrasound routinely and often for the most trivial of reasons. No one asks the question "We have the technology, we can do it, but should we do it? Or "Should we introduce it more slowly and in a way which allows us to monitor any possible adverse effects?"

It should not be forgotten that numerous studies on rats, mice and monkeys over the years have found reduced fetal weight in babies that had ultrasound in the womb compared with controls. Nor should it be forgotten that in the monkey studies quite striking behavioural differences were noticed in the babies after birth (Tarantal et al, 1993). The ultrasound babies sat or lay around the bottom of the cage, whereas the little control monkeys were up to the usual monkey tricks. Long term follow up of the monkeys has not been reported. Do they reproduce as successfully as the controls? And, let us also bear in mind, as Jean Robinson has noted: "Monkeys do not learn to read, write, multiply, sing opera, or play the violin". Human children do, and perhaps we should consider seriously whether the increases in children with dyslexia, learning difficulties and behavioural problems are related to ultrasound exposure in the womb. Furthermore, when a woman is scanned her baby's ovaries and life-time supply of eggs are also scanned. So if the woman had seven scans during her pregnancy, when her daughter eventually turns up years later at the antenatal clinic, her developing baby will already have had seven scans.

Since the introduction of ultrasound this technology has developed rapidly. Because of the wide variation in machines and the different types of ultrasound risks or claims of safety from different studies, at different times and different places are not comparable. It is not like giving a standard dose of a drug in different trials.

Despite almost thirty years of vigorous ultrasound promotion very few follow-up studies have been done on the children who were exposed in the womb. By the time that research is available the old equipment to which those children were exposed are no longer in use and have been replaced by machines that are much more powerful.

Unfortunately an unexposed population no longer exists throughout the developed world. So we have no point for comparison.

Do women really know what they consent to when they rush to the hospital to have their first routine ultrasound scan, and then trustingly agree to yet more? Before consenting to any scan the woman should be told what the purpose of this particular scan is. A consent form should be completed and signed every time an ultrasound examination is undertaken."

Reprinted with kind permission from Beverley A Lawrence Beech and Midwifery Today, All Rights Reserved, Issue 51, Autumn 1999, www.midwiferytoday.com. Beverley A. Lawrence Beech is a researcher, writer and speaker. She is honorary chair of the Association for Improvements in the Maternity Services, (AIMS), and can be contacted through www.aims.org.uk.

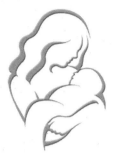

# Chapter Four - Fourth Month

Motherhood will enable you to experience every aspect of who you are as a woman. You may find this experience the most challenging and rewarding position of your life.

Pregnancy affects your entire body and most of its functions. Don't be fooled into thinking that the only thing that changes is your tummy size.

Make sure your health team is available to talk to you about any aspect of pregnancy and childbirth. Pregnancy is not the time to be embarrassed to ask important questions about your health and the health of your baby. Ask questions. Being pregnant is at times confusing. Your health team will be able to tell you how your body will react to various things at various stages. No question is too small or stupid. Second or third pregnancies may be very different from the first.

Are you are having trouble getting your current OB to talk to you, answer your questions, make eye contact with you or smile at you? Think you may have to switch at this point? If you feel that you are getting an impersonal, assembly-line practice or that your birth plan may not be complied with, remember that it is never too late to switch. One mother switched her doctor four days past her due date and another mother changed her doctor during labor.

Arrange now for a caregiver and a backup caregiver to assist you when you bring your new baby home. Many mothers feel that just getting through their pregnancy is the hard part; in reality the first thirty days after the birth of your child will continue to bring tremendous demands on your body and your hormonal system. Make sure you have the support necessary to heal completely from the birth when you bring your baby home. In many societies the mothers rest and are cared for by their families for forty days after the birth of a child.

# The Woman's Herb -
# The Remarkable Raspberry Leaf Tea

Although many people display allergic symptoms to strawberries, few cannot indulge in the fruit that ripens in the hottest part of the summer, the raspberry. The fruit is lovely, but the healthful properties in the leaves and root bark are so valuable, raspberry is known as the "Woman's Herb."

Raspberry is a relative of the rose, famous for vitamin C in the rose hip. Raspberry leaves are rich in citric acid, malic acid, tartaric acid, citrate, malate and tartarate of iron, potassium and calcium, calcium and potassium chloride, sulphate and phosphate, pectin, fragrine, vitamins A, B, C, E and fructose. The action is astringent, tonic, refrigerant, parturient, hemostatic, anti-septic, anti-abortient, anti-gonorrheal, anti-leucorrheal and anti-malarial.

Regular drinking throughout pregnancy strengthens and tones tissues, helping contractions and checks hemorrhage during labor. A perfectly safe drink, unlike black tea or coffee, raspberry leaf tea also enriches milk and helps prevent miscarriage. Raspberry leaf tea has helped with painful menstruation and lessens an overabundant period.

At menopause the adrenals are geared to take over as the ovaries gradually cease functioning. Many menopausal symptoms are caused by exhausted adrenals. Men with exhausted adrenals are well-advised to drink this tea as well.

Red raspberry leaf tea with red clover, one or more cups daily for several months, promotes fertility in men and women, prevents postnatal depression and hypertension. Pour one cup boiling water over a teaspoon of dried leaves and let it steep at least 15 minutes. Drink and heal.

# Ambivalence

Some women are ambivalent about the baby they are carrying up until the last moment of their pregnancy. This doesn't have to be you. Your baby feels this emotion, and all other emotions you have while your baby is in your womb. This is the time to make up your mind about your pregnancy and to decide that you will do your best. Occasional thoughts of whether you have made the right decision will surface from time to time: this is normal. If these thoughts are constantly with you, review the reasons why you decided to have your baby.

Be confident in your decision and in your ability to mother, even if you are not having strong maternal feelings at this time. An excellent book on emotions during pregnancy is Transformation through Birth by Claudia Panuthos. If you are feeling continually sad or hopeless about your pregnancy for any reason, seek professional help and advice, you may be at risk for prenatal or postnatal depression.

# Exercise During Pregnancy

Moderately exercising throughout your entire pregnancy will help you to keep your energy up and the extra weight down. Walking is still one of the best forms of exercise for a pregnant woman. A regular walking routine at your favorite time of day strengthens your thighs and hips, helping you to have an easier childbirth.

Regular exercise will also help you to deal with the emotional lows and highs of pregnancy and will give you the extra strength you will need for natural delivery of your baby. If you have never exercised before your pregnancy, start slowly and always stop before you are panting with exertion. Regular exercise will also improve your appearance and posture.

Regular exercise during your pregnancy can help you to have an easier labor and delivery. Walking helps your baby to turn easily in your womb to a good head-down position for a gentle delivery.

If you enjoy the water, specially designed water fitness classes for pregnancy can be found at most pools. Check out your city's Y.W.C.A.

There are specially designed exercise programs for pregnancy and a quick trip to the library will show you how to add something new to your exercise program while you are pregnant. Check with your health team before you begin.

## Rules for Exercise in Each Trimester

As your body changes and your baby develops over the nine months, what you can and can't do in terms of exercise changes too. The major benefits of postnatal exercise include: A faster recovery and healing process after giving birth, an increase in your metabolism and a faster return to your pre-pregnancy shape and fitness levels, reducing your stress levels and decreasing the likelihood of developing postnatal depression and more energy to deal with your new role as a mother. Read on to discover the specific rules you should follow in each trimester.

### First Trimester

- If you're a regular exerciser, continue with your normal exercise program.

If you're a beginner, start some form of gentle exercise like daily walks.
- You can continue to do sit-ups and curl-ups as your baby is still in the pelvic region. You should stop, though, when your tummy pops out, usually at around twelve to fourteen weeks.
- Start to do abdominal and pelvic floor exercises and work on good posture. Invest in a sports bra and a good pair of trainers.
- Listen to your body - don't exercise if you're feeling sick or tired, or have sore breasts.
- Don't get too hot when exercising.

### Second Trimester
- Avoid lying on your back after sixteen weeks.
- Slow your activity, but enjoy the feel-good factor that comes with the second trimester. Again, listen to your body.
- Most sporting bodies bar pregnant women from taking part beyond the second trimester.
- Regular participants in ball games, like tennis or netball should stop now.
- Stop using the rower at the gym. You should also stop body pump and body combat classes, and avoid circuit training.

### Third Trimester
- If you haven't already done so, switch to low-impact exercise.
- It's vital to work on posture and continue to work your abdominal muscles. And don't forget your pelvic floor exercises - if you do nothing else at this time, continue with this.
- Get measured for a new sports bra. Invest in a support belt if the weight of your baby is uncomfortable when you exercise.
- Continue mind/body classes and working out in the water. If you're a regular exerciser, follow the guidelines for your chosen activity.
- Now is the time to really abide by the golden rules, listen to your body.

Always consult your health care practitioner before beginning any exercise program.

# Sex and Pregnancy

With a normal pregnancy, you can keep having sex right up until your water breaks. Check with your doctor or midwife first if you've been treated for premature labor or if you're having any problems with your pregnancy, such as a shortened or dilated cervix, leaking amniotic fluid, placenta previa or bleeding, or if you have a history of miscarriages. There are some instances when you should avoid having sex.

As long as your pregnancy is normal, you won't hurt the baby by making love. The thick mucus plug that seals the cervix helps guard against infection. The amniotic sac and the strong muscles of the uterus also protect your baby. Though your baby may thrash around a bit after orgasm, it's because of your pounding heart, not because he knows what's happening or is feeling pain.

Sex during pregnancy can feel even better for some women, not as good for others. Increased blood flow to the pelvic area can cause engorgement of the genitals and heighten the sensation. But the same engorgement gives other women an uncomfortable feeling of fullness after intercourse ends. Also, some women may have abdominal cramps during or after intercourse. Your breasts may become enlarged and can be more tender, which can cause discomfort when they're fondled. You may have more vaginal discharge or moistness, which can make sex either more pleasurable or can result in some vaginal irritation.

If you notice a sudden change in the amount of vaginal discharge or a foul or unusual odor, check with your health practitioner. You could have a vaginal infection or your water may have broken. When your water breaks, you may feel a slow leak rather than a gush of fluid all at once.

The big changes in your body are bound to change your sex life. Some women, finally free from worries about conception and contraception, feel sexier than ever. But others are just too tired or nauseated to make love, especially in the first trimester. The second trimester is often marked by a resurging libido. Your desire may wane again in the third trimester as birth, labor, and your belly loom large, or you may simply feel unattractive or tired.

Most people find their pregnant partner as attractive as ever. But your partner's desire may be dampened by concerns for your health and the baby's, apprehension about the burdens of parenthood, fear that sex can hurt the baby, or even self-consciousness about making love in the presence of your unborn child.

Oral sex won't harm you or your baby, provided you're in a monogamous relationship where both you and your partner are HIV-negative. In fact many consider it a nice substitute if intercourse is deemed too risky.

Here are some time-tested positions and tips for making love while you're pregnant:
- Lie sideways. Having your partner on top demands increasingly creative gymnastics as your tummy swells. But lying partly sideways allows your

partner to keep most of his weight off your uterus.

- Use the bed as a prop. Your bulge isn't an obstacle if you lie on your back at the side or foot of the bed with your knees bent, and your bottom and feet perched at the edge of the mattress. Your partner can either kneel or stand in front of you.
- Lay side-by-side in the spoon position, which allows for only shallow penetration. Deep thrusts can become uncomfortable as the months pass.
- Get on top of your partner. It puts no weight on your abdomen and allows you to control the depth of penetration.

Have faith - where there's a will, there's a way. With a little experimenting, you and your partner are sure to find a technique that works for both of you.

## Shopping Tips

Find a maternity shop that rents clothing for the office and special occasions. Look for an elegant, formal outfit that you may need to wear in the months to come. Dark, solid colors without prints, patterns or buttons will make you feel less conspicuous, and you will look and feel more elegant.

During your last trimester your feet may swell. Buy any new shoes at least a half size larger with room to stretch. Purchase a blazer or suit jacket in a size two or three sizes larger than you usually wear. Make sure that you purchase the jacket in a solid color so that you can wear it with most of your outfits. You may be able to wear this for many months and it will help you feel more put together when you dress for work or the office.

### What You Need To Know Before You Have Your Baby: Ten Steps of the Mother-Friendly Childbirth Initiative

"To receive CIMS, the Coalition for Improving Maternity Services designation as "mother-friendly," a hospital, birth center, or home birth service must carry out our philosophical principles by fulfilling the Ten Steps of Mother-Friendly Care:

A mother-friendly hospital, birth center, or home birth service offers all birthing mothers:

Unrestricted access to the birth companions of her choice, including fathers, partners, children, family members, and friends;

Unrestricted access to continuous emotional and physical support from a skilled woman-for example, a doula or labor-support professional:

**Access to professional midwifery care.**

Provides accurate descriptive and statistical information to the public about its practices and procedures for birth care, including measures of interventions and outcomes.

Provides culturally competent care -- that is, care that is sensitive and responsive to the specific beliefs, values, and customs of the mother's ethnicity and religion.

Provides the birthing woman with the freedom to walk, move about, and assume the positions of her choice during labor and birth (unless restriction is specifically required to correct a complication), and discourages the use of the lithotomy (flat on back with legs elevated) position.Has clearly defined policies and procedures for: collaborating and consulting throughout the perinatal period with other maternity services, including communicating with the original caregiver when transfer from one birth site to another is necessary; linking the mother and baby to appropriate community resources, including prenatal and post-discharge follow-up and breastfeeding support.

Does not routinely employ practices and procedures that are unsupported by scientific evidence, including but not limited to the following:

- shaving;
- enemas;
- IVs (intravenous drip);
- withholding nourishment;
- early rupture of membranes;
- electronic fetal monitoring;

Other interventions are limited as follows:

- Has an induction rate of 10% or less;
- Has an episiotomy rate of 20% or less, with a goal of 5% or less;
- Has a total cesarean rate of 10% or less in community hospitals, and 15% or less in tertiary care (high-risk) hospitals;
- Has a VBAC (vaginal birth after cesarean) rate of 60% or more with a goal of 75% or more.

Educates staff in non-drug methods of pain relief and does not promote the use of analgesic or anesthetic drugs not specifically required to correct a complication.

Encourages all mothers and families, including those with sick or premature newborns or infants with congenital problems, to touch, hold, breastfeed, and care for their babies to the extent compatible with their conditions.

Discourages non-religious circumcision of the newborn.

Strives to achieve the WHO-UNICEF "Ten Steps of the Baby-Friendly Hospital Initiative" to promote successful breastfeeding:

Have a written breastfeeding policy that is routinely communicated to all health care staff;

Train all health care staff in skills necessary to implement this policy;

Inform all pregnant women about the benefits and management of breastfeeding;

Help mothers initiate breastfeeding within a half-hour of birth;

Show mothers how to breastfeed and how to maintain lactation even if they should be separated from their infants;

Give newborn infants no food or drink other than breast milk unless medically indicated;

Practice rooming in: allow mothers and infants to remain together 24 hours a day;

Encourage breastfeeding on demand;

Give no artificial teat or pacifiers (also called dummies or soothers) to breastfeeding infants;

Foster the establishment of breastfeeding support groups and refer mothers to them on discharge from hospitals or clinics.

Reprinted with kind permission of The Coalition for Improving Maternity Services(CIMS). For further information about The Coalition for Improving Maternity Services contact www.motherfriendly.org.

# What You Need To Know Before You Have Your Baby: The Risks of Cesarean Delivery to Mother and Baby

The Coalition for Improving Maternity Services (CIMS) is concerned about the dramatic increase and ongoing overuse of cesarean section. Every year since 1983 no fewer than one in five American women has given birth via major abdominal surgery. Today one in four or 25% of women have a cesarean for the birth of their baby. The rate for first-time mothers may approach one in three. Studies show that the cesarean rate could safely be halved. The World Health Organization recommends no more than a 15% cesarean rate. With a million women having cesarean sections every year, this means that 400,000 to 500,000 of them were unnecessary.

No evidence supports the idea that cesareans are as safe as vaginal birth for mother or baby. In fact, the increase in cesarean births risks the health and well being of childbearing women and their babies.

For elective repeat cesarean, the consensus of dozens of studies totaling tens of thousands of women is that elective repeat cesarean section is riskier for the mother and not any safer for the baby. Recent studies used to conclude otherwise are both seriously flawed and have been misrepresented in the media.In addition to the hazards of cesarean section per se, the risks of certain complications increase with accumulating surgeries. Studies also show that with a history of previous cesarean, seven out of ten women or more who are allowed to labor without undue restrictions will give birth vaginally, thus ending their exposure to the dangers of cesarean section.

## Hazards of Cesarean Section to the Mother

Women run 5 to 7 times the risk of death with cesarean section compared with vaginal birth.

Complications during and after the surgery include surgical injury to the bladder, uterus and blood vessels (2 per 100), hemorrhage (1 to 6 women per 100 require a blood transfusion), anesthesia accidents, blood clots in the leg (6 to 20 per 1000), pulmonary embolism (1 to 2 per 1000), paralyzed bowel (10 to 20 per 100 mild cases, 1 in 100 severe), and infection (up to 50 times more common).

One in ten women report difficulties with normal activities two months after the birth, and one in four report pain at the incision site as a major problem. One in fourteen still report incisional pain six months or more after delivery.

Twice as many women require re-hospitalization as women having normal vaginal birth.

Especially with unplanned cesarean section, women are more likely to experience negative emotions, including lower self-esteem, a sense of failure, loss of control and disappointment. They may develop postpartum depression or post-traumatic stress syndrome. Some mothers express dominant feelings of fear and anxiety about their cesarean as long as five years later.

Women having cesarean sections are less likely to decide to become pregnant again.

As is true of all abdominal surgery, internal scar tissue can cause pelvic pain, pain during sexual intercourse and bowl problems.

Reproductive consequences compared with vaginal birth include increased infertility, miscarriage, placenta previa (placenta overlays the cervix), placental abruption (the placenta detaches partially or completely before the birth), and premature birth. Even in women planning repeat cesarean, uterine rupture occurs at a rate of 1 in 500 versus 1 in 10,000 in women with no uterine scar.

## Hazards of Cesarean Section to the Baby

Especially with planned cesarean, some babies will inadvertently be delivered prematurely, Babies born even slightly before they are ready may experience breathing and breastfeeding problems.

One to two babies per 100 will be cut during the surgery.

Studies comparing elective cesarean section or cesarean section for reasons unrelated to the baby with vaginal birth find that babies are 50% more likely to have low Apgar scores, 5 times more likely to require assistance with breathing, and 5 times more likely to be admitted to intermediate or intensive care.

Babies born after elective cesarean section are more than four times as likely to develop persistent pulmonary hypertension compared with babies born vaginally. Persistent pulmonary hypertension is life threatening.

Mothers are more likely to have difficulties forming an attachment with the infant. This may be because women are less likely to hold and breastfeed their infants after birth and have rooming in and because of the difficulties of caring for an infant while recovering from major surgery.

Babies are less likely to be breastfed. The adverse health consequences of formula feeding are numerous and can be severe.

## Hazards of Elective Repeat Cesarean Section

Elective cesarean section carries twice the risk of maternal death compared with vaginal birth.

Old scar tissue increases the likelihood of surgical injury.

One more woman in every 100 with a history of more than one cesarean will have an ectopic pregnancy (embryo implants outside the womb). Hemorrhage associated with ectopic pregnancy is one of the leading causes of maternal death in the US.

Compared with women with no uterine scar, women have more than 4 times the risk of placenta previa with one prior cesarean, 7 times the risk with two to three prior cesareans, and 45 times the risk with four or more prior cesareans. Placenta previa more than doubles the chance of the baby dying and increases the rate of preterm birth more than 6 fold.

Compared with women with prior births and no previous cesareans, women with one prior cesarean or more have as much as 3 times the risk of placental abruption. With placental abruption, 6 in every 100 babies will dies, and 3 in 10 will be born too early.

The odds of placenta accreta (placenta grows into or even through the uterus) jump from 1 in 1,000 with one prior cesarean to 1 in 100 with more than one prior cesarean. Nearly all women with this complication will require a hysterectomy, nearly half will have a massive hemorrhage, and as many as 1 in 11 babies and 1 in 14 mothers will die. The incidence of placenta accreta has increased 10-fold in the last 50 years and now occurs in 1 in 2,500 births.

Women having elective repeat cesareans are more likely to experience hemorrhage requiring transfusion, blood clots and infection.

Postpartum recovery after repeat cesarean section is even more difficult when there is another child or children to care for.

Reprinted with kind permission from The Coalition for Improving Maternity Services (CIMS), a United Nations recognized NGO. CIMS is a collaborative effort of numerous individuals, leading researchers, and more than 50 organizations representing over 90,000 members. Promoting a wellness model of maternity care that will improve birth outcomes and substantially reduce costs, CIMS developed the Mother-Friendly Childbirth Initiative in 1996. A consensus document that has been recognized as an important model for improving the healthcare and well being of children beginning at birth, the Mother-Friendly Childbirth Initiative has been translated into several languages and is gaining support around the world. References for this article may be found at www.motherfriendly.org.

# What You Need To Know Before You Have Your Baby: Vaginal Birth After Cesarean - VBAC

**Q**: Is the adage "Once a cesarean, always a cesarean" true?

**A**: No, this is outdated medical thinking. There wasn't enough information available

40 years ago on the risks of labor after a cesarean birth. Also most cesareans done then were classical incisions whereas now almost all cesarean incisions are low transverse or "bikini" incisions. Studies now prove that VBAC is indeed a safer alternative to a scheduled cesarean birth for mother and baby after a low transverse uterine incision from a prior cesarean delivery.

**Q:** My doctor told me my pelvis is too small to vaginally deliver a baby over eight pounds. Is this true?

**A:** No, the pelvis and the baby's head are not fixed bone structures. During labor the pelvis opens, allowing room for the baby, whose head molds to fit. The pelvis will actually open up 33% larger than it's pre-pregnant size with a squatting position. There are several factors that contribute to this. First a hormone called relaxin is released during the latter part of pregnancy which soften the ligaments and cartilage surrounding the pelvis. Also different positions assumed during labor will change the dimensions of the pelvis such as walking, climbing stairs and squatting. This combined with the flexibility of the baby's head gives ample room for babies to move through the pelvis. The baby's head is made up of five plates that are connected with soft tissues that allow it to mold during the birth process as the baby travels through the pelvis. These bones return to their pre-birth state within hours of birth.

**Q:** I have had more than one cesarean. Is it possible for me to have a vaginal birth?

**A:** Absolutely. Studies have proven that two or more cesareans do not significantly increase the uterine rupture rate compared to having one prior cesarean in the absence of induction medication. There is a correlation however to an increase in placenta accrete with each cesarean surgery, a condition in which the placenta imbeds into the muscular layers of the uterine wall. This can cause problems with retained placenta which often results in hemorrhaging and even a hysterectomy may be needed to stop the bleeding. Another strong reason to avoid repeat cesarean births.

**Q:** My doctor says scheduling an induction will maximize my chances for a vaginal birth. What do you think?

**A:** Actually the opposite is true. Inductions as well as augmentation of labor contribute to a marked increase in uterine rupture rates and thus should be avoided if possible. Induction also leads to a higher rate of cesarean section than spontaneous labor. If an induction is medically indicated, close monitoring of mother and baby is highly recommended.

**Q:** I can't find a doctor willing to support a vaginal birth after cesarean.

**A:** Finding a doctor to be supportive can be difficult. Do not take someone's word that there is not a doctor in your area willing to support your birth. Take the time to make an appointment and go in a see several doctors and/or midwives. Ask questions and listen to their answers.

**Q:** Is it true that ACOG is recommending all women have a repeat cesarean?

**A**: No. ACOG (American College of Obstetricians and Gynecologists) says that most women with one previous cesarean delivery are candidates for VBAC and should be counseled about VBAC and offered a "trial" of labor. However, they have revised their recommendations to include that an obstetrician be immediately available during the labor of a VBAC woman.

**Q**: My baby is breech. Will I have to have a cesarean?

**A**: Not necessarily. It depends on how your baby is positioned and the experience of your doctor/midwife. With a skilled caregiver a breech vaginal delivery can be as safe or safer to mother and baby as a cesarean birth. Turning the baby is the best way to avoid a cesarean however and there are many techniques available to turn breech babies to a vertex, or head down, position.

**Q**: Doesn't a vaginal birth cause problems like pelvic floor "damage"?

**A**: Lead researcher Dr. Alastair MacLennan in an interview with Reuters Health states, "80% of the problems a woman having a vaginal delivery has, also happen to a woman having a Cesarean section." Most often it is the interventions like episiotomies, vacuum and forceps deliveries that contribute to urinary and fecal incontinence, uterine prolapse, and pelvic floor damage rather than the vaginal birth itself. Women who have had cesarean deliveries also experience urinary and fecal incontinence and other concerns due to the surgery or simply as a result of the hormones of pregnancy and/or the drugs used during the delivery.

**Q**: Wouldn't a cesarean be safer than a vaginal birth after a cesarean?

**A**: A cesarean section is major abdominal surgery with all that entails. The surgery itself, as opposed to medical problems that might lead to a cesarean increases the risk of maternal death, hysterectomy, hemorrhage, infection, blood clots, damage to blood vessels, urinary bladder and other organs, postpartum depression, post traumatic stress syndrome, and rehospitalization for complications. Potential chronic complications from scar tissue adhesions include pelvic pain, bowel problems, and pain during sexual intercourse. Scar tissue makes subsequent cesareans more difficult to perform, increasing the risk of injury to other organs as well as placenta previa, placenta accreta, infertility, ectopic pregnancy, uterine rupture in subsequent pregnancies and the risk of chronic problems from adhesions. There are also risks to the baby such as respiratory distress syndrome, prematurity, lower birth weights, jaundice, lower APGAR scores (APGAR is the means of assessing the health status of a newborn), and finally in 1 to 9 percent of cases the baby is scarred or even maimed by the scalpel.

**Q**: What is the real percentage risk of uterine rupture?

**A**: This is a difficult question because there are many factors that attribute to uterine rupture. It is widely accepted thought that for a woman who has had one previous lower transverse cesarean, the risk is 0.7% or 7 in 1000 women. If a woman has had two or more prior lower transverse cesareans her risk only increases slightly. Induction or augmentation will however increase the risk dramatically from 0.7% to 5%, and with a classical or T-incision the risk is found to be between 3% and 5%.

**Q**: Can I have a VBAC if I have a classical incision?

**A**: The reason VBAC isn't recommended with a classical incision is that it is believed that the rupture rates are higher (3-5% vs. less than 1%). However, we don't have reliable stats since women with classical incisions aren't allowed in VBAC studies. An interesting note is that in many VBAC studies, women with "unknown" incisions (lack of records) were allowed in the studies. Their inclusion did not affect the results (which indicates that rupture with a classical incision is lower than they estimate).

**Q**: When is a cesarean absolutely necessary?

**A**: • Complete placenta previa at term.
• Transverse lie
• Prolapsed cord.
• Abrupted Placenta.
• Eclampsia or severe preeclampsia with failed induction of labor.
• Large uterine tumor which blocks the cervix
• True fetal distress confirmed with a fetal scalp sampling or biophysical profile
• True cephalopelvic disproportion (CPD- baby too large for pelvis). This is extremely rare and only associated with a pelvic deformity (or an incorrectly healed pelvic break).
• Initial outbreak of active herpes at the onset of labor.
• Uterine rupture"

Reprinted with kind permission of the International Cesarean Awareness Network, Inc. All right reserved. To obtain further information visit their excellent website at www.ican-online.org.

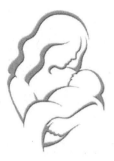

# Chapter Five - Fifth Month

Be prepared for many new emotions and dreams. Hormonal fluctuations will affect every aspect of your emotions. When you feel like crying, cry. If you find your anger surfacing use it to move forward with your life. Explain your feelings, as they come up, to your baby if you like. It is also comforting to talk them out with your partner and friends.

Make fruit your bedtime snack. You will find that fruit will satisfy your appetite and your need for extra nutrition. Fruit adds fiber, quenches your thirst, and will help you to have fewer trips to the bathroom during the night.

Read the breastfeeding section in this book during this month. Go to the library and watch breastfeeding videos. The more you know about breastfeeding now, the easier you will breastfeed your baby. Plan to attend a breastfeeding clinic in your eighth or ninth month of pregnancy so that you know where it is.

Call the La Leche number listed in the Childbirth Resource Directory to find a breastfeeding support group right in your neighborhood. You will be welcomed with open arms while you are pregnant and after. In the support group you will hear of common challenges in breastfeeding and common solutions. Often any challenges can be cleared up with a phone call or a quick meeting. Just knowing where to direct your inquiries can give you peace of mind.

If you experience pain from your stomach muscles stretching as your baby grows, lean forward while sitting to relieve the pressure on these muscles, whenever you feel the stretch.

Rock your baby in the womb. Place both hands on either side of your stomach and slowly breath in and out. You can do this first thing in the morning or last thing at night to relax both of you. Your baby will feel the soothing warmth of your hands and will always be comforted by this time together.

A woman carries her birth experience with her for rest of her life. The childbirth process is not simply a means to the end of the pregnancy. When planning your childbirth remember that this will be the most important day of your baby's life as well.

## Managing Fear of Labor and Delivery

You may have fears of labor that come up from time to time. Instead of focusing on the unknown, focus instead on the joy you will feel as you gaze into your baby's eyes and how your baby will feel against your breast as you feed your baby for the first time. Often mothers find the birth of their second child much easier than the first baby as there is less fear of the unknown. When the time comes for your child to be born nature takes over and you will be surprised at the efficiency of your body during the birth process.

Talk through your fears of pregnancy, labor and delivery and parenthood with your partner, your doctor and good friends. It will always help to ease your mind when you verbalize your concerns to others. Have faith in the natural process of childbirth, read as much as you can about childbirth, attend an informative prenatal class and plan to have professional labor support with you during your labor and delivery. Occasionally our fears are replayed in life. Decide what you are most afraid of, whether it is cesarean, dealing with pain during labor, episiotomy, stalled labor, or whatever may be concerning you personally and read everything you can on how to deal with the situation that you are most concerned with. Talk over solutions to any of your concerns with your health team.

## The Wise Women

Here are some letters from Open Season – A Survival Guide for Natural Childbirth and Vaginal Birth After Cesarean, VBAC in the 90's Nancy Wainer Cohen, on why midwives are becoming the first choice for many women in North America.

"I have an unfaltering confidence in birth, in a woman's ability to give birth, and in myself as a practitioner. No woman has ever looked in my eyes and seen doubt. This is what I love. I will always be reborn in midwifery, each day and with each birth." Meg

"You know, there is always so much more to learn. When I observed other midwives I saw them sitting on their hands and being supportive. I learn to sit on my hands, to trust, more and more each day. A woman with four previous classical cesareans wanted a homebirth. Everyone thought she was crazy and that I would be even crazier for attending her. My heart said, 'Do it. It will be fine. I always listen to my heart. It never lies to me." Mary

"Every time I saw an OB cut a woman's perineum, I felt my own was being cut. Finally I said 'No more!' I put my hand in front of the OB's knife and said, "Cut off my fingers first." Carolyn

"I have been attending births for twelve years. The most important thing I have learned is each pregnancy, labor, and birth is different. Each woman is different. Each child has its own 'journey' to make, and the mother has hers as well. I used to feel as if I was a guide. I don't think that way anymore. I am really along on the journey, too. It is a privilege to be asked along on another's sacred journey." Marie

"My message is this: Be in love with the whole process and all the people involved. Keep the wonder of it alive inside of you." Karen

"To be the best midwife I can be requires that I must be clear in mind and spirit. I must take care of my physical body–respect it. Anger and hostility interferes with the work I do. I learn, day by day, to relax and flow with birth." Pat

"I became a midwife because I had two cesareans myself. The small town where I live has a 46% c-section rate! With little education, few choices and no support, the women give in to the doctors. I have become an outspoken anti-interventionist. 98% of my mothers, and I take a lot of the so-called high-riskers; have natural deliveries." Carol

"Midwifery is definitely a calling. It's in my cells. It isn't my 'profession' it is part of me. No, it is me. There are no words to tell you the joy, the awesomeness of it all. It is a bit of heaven on this earth." Lianne

Here are some of the things that women who use midwives say about them: They are gentle; they don't injure their clients; they don't use medical interventions; they are so kind to your bottom; they aren't on a power-trip and they don't make you feel guilty or inferior or inadequate; they are patient, they know the meaning of the word "support"; they don't think the doctor's word is God; they are strong in a very loving way; they love babies!; they love women; they know how to listen; they are intuitive; they explain things; they are emotionally accessible; their hands are soft, firm and welcoming; they let me cry and complain; they are warm and compassionate; they are knowledgeable and wise; they know how to build confidence; they're very special, every one of them.

Midwives do not slap a "high-risk" label on a woman as a sentence from which there is no escape. They know steps that can be taken to reduce or eliminate risks. They do not use "gynegadgetry". Midwives often consider a woman a homebirth candidate even when many others would not: her criteria include not only the physical and the physiological, but the nutritional, emotional, psychological, sexual and spiritual, as well. In countless incidences the presence of a midwife has saved women and their babies from unnecessary surgery, unnecessary interventions, episiotomies, and from physical trauma."

## Chiropractic Care and Pregnancy

The muscle strains and back pain of pregnancy are very real and can be more than just a nuisance. The average weight gain of 25 to 35 pounds, combined with the increased stress placed on the body by the baby, can sometimes result in severe discomfort. In fact, studies have found that about half of all expectant mothers will develop low back pain at some point during their pregnancy. This is especially true during late pregnancy, when the baby's head presses down on a woman's back, legs and buttocks, putting pressure on her sciatic nerve. And for those who already suffer from low back pain, the problem can become even worse.

During pregnancy, a woman's center of gravity almost immediately begins to shift forward to the front of her pelvis and the displaced weight increases the stress on her joints. Furthermore, as the baby grows in size, the woman's weight is projected even farther forward, and the curvature of her lower back is increased, placing extra stress on her spinal disks in that area. As a result, the spine in the upper back area must compensate - and the normal curvature of her upper spine increases as well.

To combat this, during pregnancy hormones are released that help loosen the ligaments attached to the pelvic bones. But even these natural changes designed to accommodate the growing baby can result in postural imbalances, causing pregnant women to be more prone to awkward trips and falls.

### How Chiropractic Care Helps

Chiropractic care is a good alternative to over-the-counter and prescription drugs for back pain. Since a chiropractor manipulates the spine to ease back pain, there is no medication involved, making it a safe and more natural form of relief. If you are worried about the safety of the procedure, rest assured that many studies have found there to be no risk to either mother or fetus when a trained professional does spinal manipulation.

Even before you become pregnant, a chiropractor can help you out. They will be able to properly assess your body and diagnose any already existing imbalances in your pelvis or elsewhere that may increase your discomfort during pregnancy. Additionally, they will be able to detect factors in your skeletal structure that may lead to problems after you give birth.

After your pregnancy, your chiropractor can treat you to help ensure that your stretched out joints and loosened ligaments get back into their proper places. Chiropractic care may also help relieve some headaches, shoulder problems and muscle and rib discomfort caused by your changing body.

Ask your chiropractor for tips on proper back exercises and nutrition to help ensure you have a comfortable and healthy pregnancy.

### *Tips for a Healthy Back*

**Exercise**: Not only does exercise help you from gaining too much weight during your pregnancy, it also helps strengthen your muscles and prevent or relieve any discomfort you might experience. Exercising just three times a week can make a big difference in how you feel. Walking, swimming and yoga as well as using a stationary bike are all excellent forms of exercise for pregnant women. Prenatal yoga classes can especially help to relieve back tension. Always stop exercise if you experience warning signs like dizziness, nausea, blurred vision or vaginal bleeding.

**Proper Shoes**: High heels may make your legs look great but they wreak havoc on your back and posture. During pregnancy, the last thing you want is to exacerbate a backache so wear flat, comfortable shoes as often as you can. If you do have to wear high heels, go for a low heel rather than your favorite stilettos.

**Lift Properly:** Whenever you are lifting a heavy object, whether it is an older child or a large television, always bend from the knees, not your waist. It is also best not to turn your head when you lift an object. If you can, try to avoid lifting heavy objects all together when you're pregnant.

**At Work**: If you spend most of your day sitting in front of a computer, make sure your workstation is set up to be ergonomically correct. The top of your computer monitor should be no higher than eye level. Also, be sure to put your feet up on a small footrest periodically to relieve the pressure in your legs and feet. Stretch your legs by taking short walks around the office every half hour or so.

**At Home**: Get lots of rest! Don't be afraid to ask for help if you need it. Sit down and put your feet up whenever you can. If you feel tired then take a nap. When you are sleeping it is a good idea to lie on your side and place a pillow between your legs. This helps to take the pressure off of your lower back. A body pillow is very popular with many pregnant women and can be used after the baby is born to make breastfeeding more comfortable.

## Shopping Tips

Purchase a rocking chair for you and your baby. Glider rockers are an excellent investment and will last for years. A rocking chair is soothing throughout your pregnancy, great for breastfeeding and handy for those late nights after your baby arrives.

## Preventing Episiotomy

An episiotomy is a surgical cut through the perineum (the skin and tissue between the vagina and the anus) to widen the birth outlet. A number of doctors are still habitually performing this unnecessary procedure. The practice of episiotomy was initiated in the 1920s by Dr. DeLee who also popularized the "forcep" delivery which he considered the ideal form of birth. Dr. DeLee felt that episiotomies were necessary because he believed that a woman's body was not perfectly designed for childbirth. This of course is perfectly untrue.

Today's research on episiotomies, some of which has been conducted by Dr. Michael Klein, Professor of Family Medicine at the University of British Columbia shows that episiotomy can involve a woman's sense of mastery or control over her birth process. Dr. Carolyn DeMarco in her book, Taking Charge of Your Body writes, "Episiotomies can be extremely painful – even the most painful part of childbirth" and that "episiotomies are the most common cause of tears." A study by Klein found that women who have episiotomies "resumed sex later, and had more pain during sex and reported less sexual satisfaction, at least in the first three months after birth."

Henci Goer, meta-analysis childbirth researcher and author of Obstetric Myths Versus Research Realities, states, "Routine episiotomy has a ritual function but serves no medical purpose." Goer also reports on the following latest findings:

"Episiotomies do not prevent tears into or through the anal sphincter. In fact, deep tears almost never occur in the absence of an episiotomy. Even when properly repaired, tears of the anal sphincter may cause chronic problems with coital pain and gas or fecal incontinence later in life. If a woman does not have an episiotomy, she is likely to have a small tear, but with rare exceptions the tear will be at worse, no worse than a routine episiotomy. Episiotomies do not prevent urinary incontinence or improve sexual satisfaction.

"Episiotomies are not easier to repair than tears. Episiotomies do not heal better than tears. Episiotomies do not prevent birth injuries or fetal brain damage. Episiotomies increase blood loss. As with any other surgical procedure, episiotomies may lead to infection, including fatal infections. Epidurals increase the need for episiotomy. They also increase the probability of instrumental delivery. Instrumental delivery increases both the odds of episiotomy and deep tears.

The prone position during delivery increases the need for episiotomy, probably because the perineum is tightly stretched. Some techniques for reducing perineal trauma that have been evaluated and found effective are: prenatal perineal massage, slow delivery of the head, supporting the perineum, keeping the head flexed, delivering the shoulders one at a time, and doing instrumental deliveries without episiotomy."

One of the best midwife's secrets for avoiding an episiotomy is a simple, liberal application of warm oil compresses or warm water compresses applied to your perineum and around your baby's head as it begins to show. A natural tear easily heals on its own. A surgical incision will take twice as long to heal and often leads to deeper and longer tears. The perineum can be compared to a piece of cloth. It is difficult to tear a whole piece of cloth by your hands, but by making cutting a tiny cut into it with scissors the fabric tears easily all the way across. Keeping this area intact should be one of the greatest concerns of your health professionals.

During delivery you will want to stop pushing and pant as your baby's head starts to show and you feel the stretch. Unless there is some medical reason, don't let anyone rush this second stage. Slow and steady at this point will allow your baby's head to be delivered slowly, then with one shoulder out first and then the other. You need a mirror at this stage to help you to guide your pushing efforts. Your labor assistant can support your perineum by giving gentle counter pressure to your baby's head and your perineum allowing for a safe controlled delivery of the shoulders and chest and they will be carefully guiding you throughout this final stage.

Avoiding episiotomy will assist you in healing more quickly after the birth of your baby, will increase bonding with your baby and will help you to resume your sexual life with less pain and anxiety. To regain your pre-pregnancy feelings, you can tone and tighten your pelvis with your Kegel exercises after the birth of your baby. Kegel exercises and an upright and controlled delivery will all contribute to helping you avoid this unpleasant and difficult to heal optional birth intervention.

## Induced Birth – Unsafe At Any Speed

Ask your doctor about their rate of induced births and under what circumstances they would suggest induced birth. Birth is painful enough without the unnecessary stress of a forced labor. If you are planning a normal, gentle birth for your baby you will wish for your body and baby to choose the date of birth.

The drugs used to perform a birth induction are powerful and an induced birth causes both you and your baby to be at great risk. Some doctors feel it is their duty and privilege to remove your baby once you've gone 7 or 10 days past the estimated due date. Most first-time mothers easily go beyond the estimated due date with no harm to the baby or mother whatsoever if they have had a healthy pregnancy.

An induction is only indicated if you have experienced any of the following during your pregnancy: heart or kidney disease, pre-eclampsia, diabetes or high blood pressure. Should you experience any of the above you will need to look at an emergency cesarean section and perhaps even than not use the induction drugs as they will add further stress to your baby and your already stressed body. An induction must never be done for anyone's convenience, not the health team or the parents.

A due date does not have scientific validation because of the wide variation of babies and mothers. There is no way to reliably predict when your baby will be ready to be born. Some babies have easily remained in the womb for up to three and four weeks after the estimated due date. The baby was fine all along; it was the estimation of the date of birth that was wrong.

Some doctors are using ultrasounds to estimate due dates. Ultrasounds have not been proven effective in locating the due date. The further along your pregnancy; the worse the record of an ultrasound at locating an accurate due date.

Ultrasounds have also been found to be inaccurate at locating your baby's weight. The diagnosis may be that your baby is under weight, or small for gestational age and you may also be told that your placenta is aging. This can easily frighten any new mother into thinking that her baby needs to be born sooner rather than later and agreeing to a birth induction under false information.

If your baby was underweight you would want to have your baby remain in your womb for as long as possible, as long as you are having a problem-free and healthy pregnancy. Unaided, nature shows your body the exact and correct gestation for your baby. No machine or timeline can guess this exact time, when you are emotionally and physically prepared for the birth of your baby.

Should your baby at any time in a healthy pregnancy not be growing quickly enough, a simple remedy is to increase your food and liquid intake. You are nourishing your placenta every moment of the day and night and the way to increase the weight of your baby within your womb is to have small meals every two hours, during the day, thus ensuring that nutrition is continually available to you and your baby for as long as it is needed. Current research of placental aging for postmature babies has been shown to have no ill effect on the baby.

Some babies are physically incapable of existing outside of the womb. These babies cannot be saved regardless of when they leave the womb. Babies that naturally require extra time are often from larger framed parents. If your baby seems to require extra time, remember that your body knows the exact time and date that your baby will be ready. Birth is not a mystery to your body.

A great number of changes must occur within your body in order for a normal birth to happen. Changes are happening within your baby all the way up to the progression of your baby through your birth canal and the last moment when your baby takes the first breath. Normal births are between 38 and 42 weeks and longer. Birth will never be a science; it is designed by nature not man. By allowing your body to reach a natural conclusion to your pregnancy you will have a gentle and safer labor and delivery for both you and your baby.

Obtain an opinion from other medical support people if your doctor recommends induction for "any" reason. This medical intervention, often called "robbing the cradle," or "daylight obstetrics" is often done as a convenience for the hospital and staff or parents. It is better for you to take this extra time to walk, eat, relax and rest for your important upcoming position of motherhood. Your baby will appreciate this extra time for developing as well.

Henci Goer in Obstetrical Myths Versus Research Realities, reports the following findings in her meta-analysis of the latest discoveries on inductions: "Median gestational length for first-time mothers exceeds 280 days. First-time mothers have longer pregnancies than second-time mothers. Include one day to gestational length for every day the menstrual cycle normally exceeds 28 days. Healthy fetuses do not lose weight if overdue. Sonographic and clinical weight and date estimates are often wrong.

An ultrasound in the first trimester has an error of plus or minus 5 days, increasing to an error rate of plus or minus 8 days in the second trimester and further increasing to an error rate of plus or minus 22 days in the third trimester when estimating due dates. Fetal surveillance tests have high false-positive rates, often showing that there is something wrong when there really isn't. Surveillance tests do not improve outcomes and may increase risk because they lead to intervention.

Unilateral breast stimulation safely and effectively ripens the cervix and shortens pregnancy. Routine induction at any stage does not improve perinatal outcome. Inducing increases the risk of fetal distress and cesarean section, especially for first-time mothers."

She also states that "New research shows that in the absence of signs of growth retardation, and in otherwise uncomplicated pregnancies, the safest management of prolonged pregnancy is to await the spontaneous onset of labor. There is a lack of convincing evidence that the overdue fetus is at increased risk of distress or nutritional deprivation. The evidence shows that it is inappropriate to administer prostaglandins for cervical ripening for trivial reasons. The patient must be made aware of all risks of induction."

Risks of the procedure include having to be strapped to an IV or a fetal testing unit or both, causing you to be unable to move about which will slow your baby's descent. You may have accidental or forced rupturing of your membranes leaving you and your baby open to infection and cord prolapse. You will have longer, stronger and more painful contractions causing you to require drugs for pain management. You may have a prolonged labor due to drug usage and an inability to naturally push your baby out due to pain-relieving drugs.

Possible oxygen deprivation to your baby can be caused by the extremely long and hard contractions. The next step may be having your baby surgically removed with either an episiotomy with forceps or at the last stage an emergency cesarean section for fetal distress or for failure to progress should your body or baby not be ready to deliver. And so goes the chain of events.

Possible side effects from the induction procedure include post postpartum hemorrhage, uterine rupture, blood pressure problems, shock and confusion after delivery, prolonged bleeding of six weeks or more, anemia from prolonged blood loss, and possible mental and emotional disturbances, including nightmares and insomnia, and prolonged postnatal depression. Side effects to your baby may include brain damage from oxygen deprivation during labor leading to fetal distress, requiring immediate forced delivery.

Should your baby act adversely to the drug or if the induction is not timed correctly your chance of having an emergency cesarean is extremely high, over 50% in some cases. Your baby may experience cranial hemorrhage and may well become stressed before its first breath. Other risks and side effects of the drugs on the infant are yet to be studied and may include a weakened immune system leading to eczema, asthma, allergies, hives and food intolerance's in our babies.

Obstetricians are also using this dangerous drug to speed up labor. The same risks and side effects can occur to both the mother and baby. Studies are now showing that simple nipple stimulation in a stalled labor can have the same effect without any risks or side effects. Once again this is a case where an intervention is used for the convenience of the hospital staff rather than the best interests of the mother and baby.

In With Child: Birth Through the Ages, Jenny Carter and Teresa Duriez, the procedure of induction is put into context with the history of childbirth. "Artificial induction of labor was hardly a new feature of birth intervention; for centuries it has been employed either for motives of self-interest, particularly by 'granny' midwives anxious to get off home, or for medical reasons, such as preventing the mother from having to carry a large fetus. In America in the first decades of this century, it was not uncommon for labor to be hastened so that the delivery of a smaller baby would make the labor easier for the mother. There was no consideration of the possible effect on the child.

By the 1940s and 50s, however, it had become common for "fetal indication" to be taken into account when assessing the need for obstetric intervention. That is, doctors began to intervene in the birth process for the sake of the child, even if there were no signs of distress in the mother.

The active management of labor became very much a feature of modern obstetrics following the synthesis of oxytocin and the development of the prostaglandins. Emanuel Friedman in the 1950s presented computations of the average length of time taken in labor by women of various obstetrical histories. If labor did not follow the chart to the satisfaction of the obstetrician a drip was set up to speed up or slow down the process. This process is not as simple as it might sound. One of the disadvantages of using an oxytocin drip to speed up labor is that it tends to increase the strength and frequency of contractions, making pain relief more or less essential. If pethidine or a similar drug is administered to counter the pain, this will in turn slow down the contractions. In order to speed them up again, more oxytocin is given; this in turn causes greater pain and so on.

This particular type of intervention reached its height in Britain in the 1960s and early 70s when induction became not merely a means of protecting mother or fetus, but quite simply a means of achieving the convenient administration and smooth running of the hospital. In 1974, 38% of the births in England and Wales were being induced. And yet 1974 had seen widespread debate about the wisdom of a policy of wholesale induction, and an article in the Lancet in that year concluded that until unequivocal evidence is available, the public is right to question medical practices of doubtful validity that are based on convenience.

Research has now shown that there is a high incidence of fetal distress connected with large doses of oxytocin. An American study found that a slowing down of the fetal heart rate was more common in induced labors, due to a greater intensity of contractions and counter pressure on the fetal head caused by greater resistance of the birth canal. There is no predetermined correct dose of oxytocin.

By the early 1980s the fashion for induction for convenience had almost passed, certainly in Britain. There is no sure way of judging that the time is right for induction and there will inevitably be a proportion of cases in which an error in dating of gestation results in a premature child who may die or suffer irreparable damage in the neonatal period.

In Take This Book to the Obstetrician with You, Karla Morales and Charles Inlander, the authors speak about the controversial nature of inductions. "Hospitals emphasize speed and efficiency. Hospital space is limited and expensive. Every hospital service has its break-even point below which the service loses money, at which it pays for itself, and above which it makes a profit. Obstetrics is no exception. Delivery suites must reflect a high turnover rate to pay the mortgage on the first of the month and staff salaries every other Friday. From an economic point of view, hospitals cannot afford to allow women to labor at their own natural, unhurried pace.

The usual interventions employed are amniotomy to induce labor and intravenous administration of Pitocin or vaginal application of Prostin to stimulate labor. What's the problem with artificial augmentation of labor? Just ask any woman who has been given Pitocin, the common synthetic version of the hormone oxytocin. Many, if not most, will report longer and stronger contractions and shorter intervals between contractions than they experience in unstimulated labor. Thus, the stage is set for yet another intervention, in this case painkilling drugs for the relief of contractions of overwhelming intensity. As for possible adverse effects of elective stimulation of labor on the fetus, various reports relate how the strength and rapidity of contractions can decrease the ability of the fetus to restore its supply of oxygen between contractions. So the door swings open to yet another intervention, perhaps forceps delivery or a cesarean section. Ask your doctor about his percentage of induced labors. Doctors who perform inductions for medical indications only induce less than 10 percent – some less than 5 percent."

## What You Need To Know Before You Have Your Baby - Reasons to Avoid Induction of Labor

"Are your feet swollen and is your back killing you? Is sleeping upright the only way that you can manage to fall asleep between the demands of your bladder and your baby's kicking spells?

This is the life of a pregnant mother in her ninth month. The offer of a way out of this physically uncomfortable conundrum appears at first to be a blessing.

This is the seduction of induction. Let's face it, the induction of labor has become commonplace, so commonplace, in fact, that the average length of pregnancy has dropped nearly a week in most recent studies. This medical procedure may have some pretty severe downsides to both mother and baby. Before you agree to this medical procedure of induction, ask yourself and your partner the following questions:

1. Are you willing to risk having a premature baby? Occasionally labor is induced before the baby is ready. New studies show us that babies who are even slightly premature have more problems at birth and beyond, even without time in the neonatal intensive care unit.

2. Are you willing to experience a more painful labor? Due to the faster lead up to strong contractions that come on at an unnatural rate and pattern, this medical form of labor may take your body by surprise. Some also say that this is due to your baby being in a less favorable position, since he or she didn't send the "all clear" signal for labor to begin.

3. Are you ready emotionally and physically? In normal birth, labor begins on its own. You may have had ideas about how labor would begin for you. Perhaps you saw yourself making a mad dash to the hospital in the middle of the night or couldn't wait until your water broke. This can be difficult to reconcile with the reality of induction.

4. Are you willing to risk harm for you or your baby? Sometimes when labor is

induced, the baby does not tolerate the artificially strong contractions well. This can lead to fetal distress. When certain medications are used to induce labor, there is an increase in the risk of damage to the uterus in the form of uterine rupture.

5. Are you willing to have further interventions during labor and birth? This may include additional interventions to help monitor you and your baby while they use strong medications to force your cervix open or continuous fetal monitoring, rendering you unable to walk or move about. It can also include an increase in the number of forceps deliveries and the use of a vacuum extractor and an increased risk for emergency cesarean delivery. It is also possible that the induction may not work and you are then either sent home or surgically delivered via a cesarean because of the failure of the induction and the stress a failed induction will create in your body and your baby. (If the induction does not work you have a 50% chance of requiring immediate emergency cesarean delivery.)

There are times when labor induction is medically indicated. (In cases of extreme emergency, you may need to consider moving right to a cesarean delivery, and by-passing induction, if either the mother or baby is in extreme difficulty because of a medical condition. Adding the induction drugs to an already stressed mother and baby may cause additional damages to both.) Be sure to discuss these important issues with your medical support team during your prenatal visits.

Reprinted with kind permission from Robin Elise Weiss, BA, LCCE, ICCE-CPE, Copyright 2006, All Rights Reserved. Robin Elise Weiss is a mother of seven, a certified childbirth educator, doula and has attended over 500 births since 1989. Her web site, The Pregnancy Birth site at About.com has grown to be one of the largest and most well-read pregnancy sites on the Internet. Her latest book, The About.com Guide to Having A Baby is now available at www.pregnancy.about.com and www.robineliseweiss.com.

## What You Need To Know Before You Have Your Baby: Cytotec Induction and Off-Label Use

Without adequate testing of Cytotec (misoprostol) for labor induction, obstetricians simply began to use it on their birthing women. They were taking advantage of a huge loophole in our drug regulatory system. Once a drug is approved by the FDA for a specific medical indication and put on the market, there is absolutely nothing to prevent any doctor from using that drug for any indication, in any dose, for any patient he or she chooses. Since the label of the drug contains the indications approved by the FDA, this is called "off-label" use of a drug.

When obstetricians using Cytotec induction are confronted about their willingness to use a drug "off-label," they inevitably answer: "We use drugs off-label all the time." There are several serious problems with this answer. First, in reality, using Cytotec for induction is not "off-label" at all—it is "on-label contraindicated." On the Cytotec label it is explicitly written that this drug is contraindicated for use on pregnant women. Contraindication would not be on the label unless data exists suggesting possible serious risks from such use. "On-label contraindicated" is a whole different level of risk-taking than a use that is not mentioned one way or the other on the label.

A second reason to be concerned with the offhand answer of some obstetricians is that all off-label use is lumped together as though there were equal risks involved. During a case I was involved in, I asked the obstetrician about the off-label use of Cytotec for labor induction. He replied with the same answer that I have heard from so many clinicians: "We use Cytotec off-label for induction just like we use other drugs off-label all the time." Compare this to someone involved in a fatal car accident who is asked why he did not follow traffic laws and drove 100 miles an hour in a 25 mile an hour zone. The driver answers: "Traffic laws are disobeyed all the time. Why just last week there were dozens of parking tickets given out in this city." You can't compare the risks of excessive speeding with the risks of illegal parking. And you can't compare the risks of Cytotec induction with the risk involved in giving other drugs to pregnant women off-label. A survey of 731 pregnant women revealed they had been given 10 drugs while pregnant (1). But of the 10 drugs given off-label, the use of nine of them on pregnant women carried very little risk while the use of the tenth drug, the prostaglandins (including Cytotec), have proven serious risks including uterine rupture, following which one in four babies die.

Another problem with the excuse "we give drugs off-label all the time" is that the doctors using it are taking matters into their own hands when it comes to the use of drugs on their patients. They are unwilling to wait for the scientific evidence that shows whether this use of the drug is safe. This represents both a cavalier disregard for the safety of women and babies and a total lack of faith in the drug regulatory system.

Those doctors and midwives using Cytotec for induction of labor off-label need to understand that they are taking very big chances with the safety of the women and babies they serve. Just about everyone in the world, after taking a careful look at the scientific evidence, has concluded we don't yet know enough about the risks to be willing to use it. This is illustrated in the following list of organizations that do and do not recommend Cytotec (misoprostol) for labor induction:

**Recommends:**
1.  American College of Obstetricians and Gynecologists (ACOG)
**Does not recommend:**
1.  U.S. Food and Drug Administration
2.  Best scientific opinion—Cochrane Database
3.  Searle (manufacturer of Cytotec)

4. Society of Obstetricians and Gynaecologists of Canada
5. British Royal College of Obstetricians and Gynecologists
6. All obstetric organizations in Scandinavia
7. FIGO (International Federation of Gynecology and Obstetrics)
8. World Health Organization
9. Obstetric organizations and drug regulatory agencies in many other countries

How can ACOG possibly be willing to stand alone in opposition to the best scientific opinion in the world? Because so many of ACOG's members already use Cytotec induction off-label for its incredible convenience, the organization needs to support its members by recommending this practice. This means ACOG must find a paper published in a prominent U.S. journal supporting Cytotec induction. In ACOG's recommendation on Cytotec induction, the organization leans heavily on a paper by A.B. Goldberg and other authors published in the New England Journal of Medicine (2). Let's take a careful look at the contents of this paper, as it is a superb example of torturing the data until it confesses to what the authors want it to say:

"Prescribing a medication for an off-label indication is common in the treatment of pregnant women." This argument has no justification. Common usage of something does not prove it is a good idea. Experience in medical practice can often mean gaining more and more confidence in a mistake. Furthermore, as we have seen, some drugs have no serious risks involved while others carry very serious risks. And such widespread off-label prescribing is not found in other fields of medical practice.

Next, off-label use "is not considered experimental if based on sound scientific evidence." The whole purpose of on-label use is to guarantee the consumer that there is sound scientific evidence. With the off-label use of Cytotec for labor induction there are several problems:

First, no one can disagree that for a number of years in the early 1990s Cytotec was in widespread use before there was any sound scientific evidence. No one even knew what the proper dose should be and everyone was experimenting with dosage and protocol. I find no concern from ACOG or many individual obstetricians with this indisputable fact. Thousands of women were given Cytotec without knowing that it was off-label and experimental, thus giving them no opportunity for informed consent. Proof of the danger of such nonevidence-based practice came in 1999, when there was enough evidence showing the danger of Cytotec use in VBAC that even ACOG came out against it. How many women with VBAC were given Cytotec induction between 1990 and 1999? Almost certainly thousands. How many ruptured uteri? Almost certainly hundreds. How many babies died? Almost certainly dozens. How many women died? We know there were at least several. But today, rather than using this experience to push for more evidence before use, ACOG and some individual obstetricians are pushing for more use of Cytotec when its safety is still in serious doubt.

Second, who decides when there is "sound scientific evidence"? Here there is no agreement. ACOG says there is good data to support Cytotec induction. But ACOG is not a scientific body; it is an organization of professionals—a trade union trying to protect the interests of its members. The paper's authors agree with ACOG, but a careful look at their own review shows a very flimsy database on risks. They never directly say that Cytotec induction is "safe," nor do they say that we know enough about its risks. In fact, they say the opposite.

The authors greatly confuse the reader by lumping together all uses of Cytotec during pregnancy: first trimester medical abortion, induction of labor, postpartum hemorrhage. Each of these indications has very different data and should never be combined. "Two hundred studies involving a total of more than 16,000 women" is falsely inflating the data and is most misleading. The number of studies on Cytotec labor induction is far fewer. Most of them are not randomized experimental trials, and all of them, trials included, are too small to have sufficient statistical power for the less common but catastrophic risks such as uterine rupture, perinatal mortality and maternal mortality.

The paper has a section titled "Misoprostol in the Third Trimester of Pregnancy." The first part of this section is devoted to efficacy (not risk); no one is debating the effectiveness of this drug. The debate is with the risks and here the authors admit there is more "uterine hyperstimulation with associated changes in fetal heart rate" and more "meconium-stained fluid." The authors also write, "because there were so few serious adverse effects, the relative risk of rare adverse outcomes with the use of misoprostol for labor induction remains unknown." (Italics mine.) So these authors never say this drug is safe for induction and admit that with regard to risks, we don't know enough! The last paragraph in this section is a review of studies trying to find the correct dosage for Cytotec induction. Here, the authors point out that only recently has there been any kind of idea about dosage amount. This was because researchers were trying to lower one of the documented risks—uterine hyperstimulation. In this nine-page paper, there were only a few sentences about the risks of Cytotec induction. These sentences admit that the risk of adverse outcomes remains unknown. This is a very weak evidence base and can in no way be considered "sound scientific evidence."

In the section titled "Induction of Labor in Women with Previous Cesarean Section," the authors review the research showing the huge increase in risk of uterine rupture in VBAC if Cytotec induction is used and correctly conclude that it should not be used in this way. They never mention that the paper showing the risk of uterine rupture with Cytotec induction in VBAC was published in 1999, a decade after Cytotec induction had been used on large numbers of VBAC women.

In fact, because the number of cases of uterine rupture being reported was on the increase in the 1990s, ACOG responded with a recommendation that VBAC be done only in the hospital with an obstetrician and anesthesiologist at the ready. This recommendation made the organization's obstetrician members happy but was a disaster for birthing women, midwives, family physicians and small hospitals. ACOG, instead of recommending stopping Cytotec induction, recommended surrounding women having VBAC with experts to deal with the rupture when it happens. This would be like children drowning in a lake at summer camp and, instead of teaching the children to swim, the counselors put a couple of life preservers in the lake. ACOG has yet to do the obvious and demand research to monitor uterine ruptures to determine the reason for the increase and the likely relationship to Cytotec and other forms of induction.

While one paper quoted by ACOG clearly shows the increased risk of uterine rupture if prostaglandin gels are used in VBAC (3), I have been unable to find any research which looks at the contribution that Cytotec induction makes to this increase. We know that the incidence of uterine rupture has increased overall, but we do not know how Cytotec specifically factors in to this increase. The risk of uterine rupture after VBAC is 1 in 200 births, while the risk of uterine rupture with VBAC using Cytotec induction is 1 in 20 births—a tenfold increase. Because we know that the rate of induction of labor in the U.S. doubled in the 1990s, resulting in a convenient and significant increase in the rate of births Monday through Friday (4), it is quite likely that the increase in uterine rupture reported was related to the increase in induction, especially with Cytotec. Therefore, the ACOG recommendation on VBAC is not justified.

Goldberg and the other authors conclude in their paper that there is strong and consistent evidence to support the use of misoprostol for induction in the third trimester. This opinion is most inconsistent with the little data they present on the serious adverse effects (risks) of Cytotec induction. Their opinion is nevertheless used by ACOG. Because of the enormous advantages of Cytotec induction to the practicing obstetrician, the opinion is suspect. As the previous list shows, there is a large group of experts that disagrees with this opinion, believing the evidence is still insufficient to support Cytotec's use in labor induction when existing evidence gives strong indications of several serious risks. When there is disagreement on the evidence among the experts, the most conservative and safest course for the clinician to follow is the fundamental principle of medical practice: first do no harm.

Doctors find it difficult to admit mistakes. Here we have a big mistake—Cytotec induction with VBAC—that went on for years. Yet, there is no discussion of the error or what to do so it won't happen again.

Reprinted with kind permission of Marsden Wagner, MD, MS and Midwifery Today, originally published in Midwifery Today, Issue 67, Fall 2003, www.midwiferytoday.com. Marsden Wagner, born in San Francisco, his education at University of California at Los Angeles (UCLA) included an M.D., clinical specialty training in pediatrics, then in perinatology (neonatology and obstetrics) followed by two years post-graduate study with an advanced scientific degree in perinatal science. Following several years of full time clinical practice and some years as a full time faculty member at UCLA, he was a Director of Maternal and Child Health for the California State Health Department. After six years as Director of the University of Copenhagen-UCLA Health Research Center, he was for 15 years Director of Womens and Childrens Health for the World Health Organization. He is now an independent consultant. With extensive experience in maternity care in industrialized countries, including midwifery and the appropriate use of technology during pregnancy and birth, he has consulted and lectured in over 50 countries and given testimony before the US Congress, British Parliament, French National Assembly, Italian Parliament, Russian Parliament and others. His publications, in 11 different languages, include 131 scientific papers, 20 book chapters and 14 books. Dr. Wagner's latest book is called Creating Your Birth Plan - The Definitive Guide to a Safe and Empowering Birth. For more information contact his website at www.marsdenwagner.com.

# What You Need To Know Before You Have Your Baby: Problems and Hazards of Induction of Labor

The Coalition for Improving Maternity Services (CIMS) is concerned about the dramatic increase and ongoing overuse of induction of labor. The U.S. induction rate has more than doubled since 1989, rising from one woman in ten to one woman in five in 2001. This may, however, grossly undercount the true incidence of labor induction. Nearly half of women in a 2002 survey reported that some effort has been made to start labor artificially. The World Health Organization recommends no more than a 10 percent induction rate. Despite modern techniques, induction of labor still introduces considerable risk compared with natural onset of labor, and many, if not most, inductions are done for reasons that are not supported by sound medical research.

### Hazards of Labor Induction

First-time mothers have approximately twice the likelihood of cesarean section with induction compared with natural onset of labor. This risk is due to the procedure itself, not any reason that might have led to inducing labor. Inducing labor at 41 weeks in a hypothetical population of 100,000 first-time mothers will result in somewhere between 3,700 and 8,200 excess cesareans and cost an extra $29 to $39 million.

Women who have had prior vaginal births may increase their chances of cesarean section five-fold if the cervix is not ready for labor, and they are given cervical ripening agents. Inducing 100,000 hypothetical women with prior births at 41 weeks will result in between 100 and 2,300 excess cesareans and cost an extra $25 o $26 million.

All induction agents can cause uterine hyperstimulation (contractions too long, too strong, and too close together and higher baseline muscle tension). Uterine hyperstimulation can cause fetal distress. This means that, paradoxically, inducing labor because of concern over the baby's condition may cause the very problem the induction was intended to forestall while the baby might have tolerated natural labor.

Induction of labor involves the need for other interventions - IV drip, continuous electronic fetal monitoring, usually confinement to bed - that also can have adverse effects.

Rupturing fetal membranes, a routine component of labor induction, can cause fetal distress and increases the likelihood of cesarean section. It may also precipitate umbilical cord prolapse (a life-threatening emergency for the baby in which the umbilical cord slips down into the vagina). Forty percent of all full term births involving cord prolapse were induced labors, rising to nearly 50% of births involving prolapse at 42 weeks or more.

Induced labors are usually more painful, which can increase the need for epidural analgesia. Epidurals introduce a higher probability of a host of adverse effects on the labor, the baby, and the mother.

Women with prior cesarean sections have a slightly increased probability of the scar giving way with Pitocin (oxytocin) induction (8 per 1,000 vs 5 per 1,000 with spontaneous labor onset) and greatly increased risk when prostaglandins (24 per 1,000) are used for cervical ripening or induction. Prostaglandins include Cytotec (misoprostol), Prepidil (prostaglandin E2) and Cervidil (prostaglandin E2).

## Hazards and Problems of Induction Agents

### Cytotec (Misoprostol)

Cytotec, although widely used as an induction agent, is neither formulated nor intended for use in labor. Cytotec's manufacturer, Searle, has repudiated its off-label use as an induction/cervical ripening agent because of Cytotec's attendant risks.

The FDA states that Cytotec's major adverse effects include uterine hyperstimulation, which can become severe and result in profound fetal distress; uterine rupture; amniotic fluid embolism, which has a high maternal and infant mortality rate; severe genital bleeding; shock; fetal death; and maternal death. Other adverse effects include retained placenta, cesarean section, and passage of meconium (the baby's first stool) into the amniotic fluid, which can cause a type of newborn pneumonia if inhaled.

Cytotec is commonly believed to pose a life-threatening risk only in women with a uterine scar or with high doses. However, cases of maternal and infant death and hemorrhage requiring hysterectomy have been reported in women with no uterine scar, some of whom were given a minimal dose.

Cytotec dosage cannot be controlled because the drug is a small pill that must be cut into pieces.

Once given, the drug cannot be rescinded or the dosage reduced in case of adverse effects.

Cytotec does not decrease cesarean rates compared with prostaglandin E2, which is FDA-approved for use in labor.

Cytotec's only advantages compared with prostaglandin E2 are much reduced cost and faster labors. Both benefit only hospitals and doctors as short labors are usually intense, tumultuous and difficult.

### Prostaglandin E2 (Prepidil, Cervidil)

Prostaglandin E2 can cause uterine hyperstimulation and fetal distress. Fetal distress can require cesarean section.

Prostaglandin E2 does not reduce excess cesareans associated with labor induction.

Unless the drug is formulated in a tampon (Cervidil), the drug cannot be rescinded or the dosage reduced in case of adverse effects.

### Oxytocin (Pitocin)

Complications of oxytocin (Pitocin) include uterine hyperstimulation, which can lead to fetal distress; twice the chance of the baby being born in poor condition, postpartum hemorrhage and greater probability of newborn jaundice. Rare, severe, maternal complications include uterine rupture and water intoxication leading to coma and death. Oxytocin may also cause brain damage or death in the baby.

### Medical Research Fails to Support Common Induction Rationales

Elective induction of labor, that is, induction for non-medical reasons such as convenience, exposes babies and mothers to the hazards of induction with no counterbalancing benefit.

Inducing labor for suspected big baby produces no benefits but increases the likelihood of cesarean section.

No credible evidence supports inducing labor in women with gestational - as opposed to pre-existing - diabetes.

Routinely inducing labor for prelabor rupture of membranes does not reduce the incidence of newborn infection with the exception of women testing positive for Group B strep who do not receive IV antibiotics during labor.

Inducing labor in women with Group B strep has not been shown to improve outcomes when antibiotics are given regardless of membrane status and is not part of the Centers for Disease Control recommended guidelines.

Studies claiming to support routine induction of labor at 41 weeks of pregnancy have serious flaws. No research supports routine induction at any earlier point in pregnancy; no sound research supports routine induction at any point in pregnancy.

Proponents of inducing labor at full-term argue that the stillbirth rate and the rates of other newborn complications increase markedly after that date, but, in fact, these rates show no such increase. Induction at 41 weeks in a hypothetical population of 100,000 first-time mothers would theoretically prevent 120 fetal deaths that would statistically occur in the ensuing week, but:

We don't know how many of those deaths would actually be prevented by routine induction in that they were unpredictable events in healthy mothers carrying healthy, normally formed babies.

That number would be offset by some babies dying as a result of the hazards of induction.

Any decrease in fetal deaths would be outweighed by the infertility, miscarriage, and fetal and newborn losses consequent to the excess cesareans.

Forty-one weeks is the median length of pregnancy in healthy first-time mothers. This means that one-half of such pregnancies will last longer than 41 weeks.

If there is no reason to curtail the natural length of pregnancy, then there is no reason for measures such as stripping or sweeping membranes, which themselves introduce the possibility of risk."

The Coalition for Improving Maternity Services (CIMS), a United Nations recognized NGO, is a collaborative effort of numerous individuals, leading researchers, and more than 50 organizations representing over 90,000 members. Promoting a wellness model of maternity care that will improve birth outcomes and substantially reduce costs, CIMS developed the Mother-Friendly Childbirth Initiative in 1996. A consensus document that has been recognized as an important model for improving the healthcare and well being of children beginning at birth, the Mother-Friendly Childbirth Initiative has been translated into several languages and is gaining support around the world. For further information on this initiative contact www.motherfriendly.org.

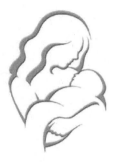

# Chapter Six - Sixth Month

Drink extra water. Keep a glass beside you at your desk and sip on it during the day. Remember you are flushing the waste of two people now. Do not hold your urine in when you need to go as this can cause bladder and kidney infections. Your bladder holds a smaller amount now, so you must adjust for that by urinating more frequently.

Do not lie flat on your back. Always lie on your side, preferably your left side, to avoid constricting your blood flow and oxygen to your baby. This includes during your prenatal visits, sleeping, and of course avoid lying on your back at any time during your labor and delivery.

## Natural Remedies for Heartburn

If you find yourself a victim of heartburn, before reaching for the Tums or Maalox, look to your diet. Eat plenty of raw food with each meal. Plan to eat only raw fruits and vegetable for one day to re-establish your digestive enzymes to break the cycle of heartburn. Make sure each meal contains raw fruits or vegetables. You can also buy digestive enzymes at the health food store and take them with every meal.

Eat your largest meal earlier in the day. Snack on fruit or vegetables in the early evening. Celery is a great antidote if heartburn strikes during the evening when you are out. Make sure to chew the fruit or vegetables well to release the enzymes.

When sleeping, you may want to arrange your pillows so that you are in a semi-reclining position.

Avoid foods that are fatty or greasy. Foods that are too acidic or too spicy may also bother you. Stay away from carbonated drinks, processed meats and junk foods.

Avoid using antacids that contain aluminum or bicarbonate of soda.

These can interfere with absorption of certain nutrients, upset your acid base balance and possibly harm your baby.

Calcium in the form of pills, powder or liquid is a natural antacid and can be used in doses of up to 1,200 mg per day. Magnesium should always be taken with calcium at about half the dosage of the calcium.

One teaspoon of slippery elm bark powder which is found in health food stores mixed with honey or hot water neutralizes stomach acidity and soothes the stomach.

When you travel, you can carry raw almonds and chew on them slowly to help relieve heartburn.

## Natural Remedies for Muscle Cramping

Keep pillows under your knees or feet to reduce cramping while you are sleeping. If you get a bad cramp during the night flex your toes and feet forward while still lying down to stretch those muscles. Rotate your ankles. If the cramp is really strong, stand up and put your weight on it.

Drinking more water during the day will help to ease evening leg cramps. Calcium tablets have also been found to help relieve cramping.

## Prenatal Classes

Start looking for an independent childbirth instructor now. Some hospital supported prenatal classes promote the various medical interventions offered at their hospital. The best value for your money is an independent instructor who will talk to you about avoiding unnecessary medical interventions, natural pain relief methods, and the emotional and spiritual aspects of birth. The more knowledge you acquire about the birth process the faster and easier your labor and delivery will be. Take a partner, if you have one, if not go alone.

Many prenatal courses are available over a weekend or a couple of weekdays. Ask for referrals from your health team to find the best class. Each class will have its own ideas or philosophies about the birth process, interview the instructors to see if their ideas match yours. Read your birth plan over the telephone to make sure they have experience in the birth you want for your baby. Look in the Childbirth Resource Directory located in this guide for referrals on independent childbirth educators in your city.

## Home Engineering

If at this point you are feeling large and awkward and wondering how you are going to get your house cleaned, set up a plan for yourself. It may just seem like too much of an effort all at once and it is. Try doing one or two things each day. For example, dust on Monday, wash sheets and towels on Tuesday, have someone else vacuum on Wednesday, sweep and mop the floor on Thursday, do the bathrooms on Friday, clean the kitchen on Saturday, and do laundry on Sunday! Keeping things as tidy as possible and 'put away' each day also helps. Your home may not be all clean all at the same time, but each job gets done in turn. Hire someone to mow your lawn or shovel your sidewalk. You will find that once your baby arrives, the same principles apply.

Keep your good humor! Things can and will go wrong when you become a new size. Realize that simple tasks may become difficult either because of your increasing size or because of your preoccupation. You will forget things and you may be unable to manage some tasks that were part of your everyday routine. So, when you burn supper or forget to return a phone call or can't reach that top shelf in the kitchen cabinets, remember these are short-term challenges you can shrug off.

## What You Need To Know Before You Have Your Baby: Optimum Fetal Positioning

"'**Optimal Fetal Positioning**' is a theory developed by midwife, Jean Sutton, who found that the mother's position and movement could influence the way her baby lay in the womb in the final weeks of pregnancy. Many difficult labors result from malpresentation, where the baby's position makes it hard for the head to move through the pelvis, so changing the way the baby lies could make birth easier for mother and child.

The 'occiput anterior' position is ideal for birth - it means that the baby is lined up so as to fit through your pelvis as easily as possible. The baby is head down, facing your back, with his back on one side of the front of your tummy. In this position, the baby's head is easily 'flexed', his chin tucked onto his chest, so that the smallest part of his head will be applied to the cervix first. The diameter of his head which has to fit through the pelvis is approximately 9.5 cm, and the circumference approximately 27.5cm. The position is usually 'Left Occiput Anterior' or LOA - occasionally the baby may be Right Occiput Anterior or ROA.

The 'occiput posterior' (OP) position is not so good. This means the baby is still head down, but facing your tummy. Mothers of babies in the 'posterior' position are more likely to have long and painful labors as the baby usually has to turn all the way round to facing the back in order to be born. He cannot fully flex his head in this position, and diameter of his head which has to enter the pelvis is approximately 11.5cm, circumference 35.5cm.

This means that often posterior babies do not engage (descend into the pelvis) before labor starts. The fact that they don't engage means that it's harder for labor to start naturally, so they are more likely to be 'late'. Braxton-Hicks contractions before labor starts may be especially painful, with lots of pressure on the bladder, as the baby tries to rotate while it is entering the pelvis. Posterior presentation is more of a problem for first babies and their mothers than it is for subsequent births; when a mother has given birth before; there is generally much more room for maneuvering, so it is easier for the baby to rotate during labor.

The rate of posterior presentation has increased drastically in the last few decades, possibly in line with changes in the way women use their bodies. Sitting in car seats and leaning back on comfortable sofas, together with less physical work, have combined to produce an increase in posterior presentations. Paying attention to your posture in the last few weeks of pregnancy can help to reverse this trend. Since keeping reasonably active in pregnancy, and practicing good posture, isn't going to do anyone any harm, this theory deserves to be considered.

## When do you need to start doing something about this?

Pay attention to your posture at the time when your baby may be starting to 'engage', which means its head will be descending into the pelvis. This means for the last six weeks of your first pregnancy, and the last two or three weeks of subsequent pregnancies. In your second and later pregnancies, the uterus is roomier and the baby will not normally start to descend into the pelvis until later and often not until labor starts.

## What position is your baby in?

This is important because you need to know when your baby moves into a good position, so that you can encourage it to stay there! You can learn to tell what position your baby is in, by asking midwives to show you what to look out for, and by practicing feeling for the baby yourself.

When the baby is anterior, the back feels hard and smooth and rounded on one side of your tummy, and you will normally feel kicks under your ribs. Your belly button (umbilicus) will normally poke out, and the area around it will feel firm. When the baby is posterior, your tummy may look flatter and feel squashier, and you may feel arms and legs towards the front, and kicks on the front towards the middle of your tummy. The area around your belly button may dip in to a concave, saucer-like shape. If you feel the baby move, try to work out what body part was moving. Remember that heads feel hard and round, while bottoms feel soft and round! It may take a lot of concentration and trying to work things out at first, but you soon get the hang of it.

If your baby is posterior, you may find that you suffer backache during late pregnancy (of course, many women suffer backache then anyway). You may also experience long and painful 'practice contractions' as your baby tries to turn around in order to engage in the pelvis.

## Practical steps to avoid posterior positions

The baby's back is the heaviest side of its body. This means that the back will naturally gravitate towards the lowest side of the mother's abdomen. So if your tummy is lower than your back, for example, you are sitting on a chair leaning forward, then the baby's back will tend to swing towards your tummy. If your back is lower than your tummy, for example, you are lying on your back or leaning back in an armchair, then the baby's back may swing towards your back.

Avoid positions that encourage your baby to face your tummy. The main culprits are said to be lolling back in armchairs, sitting in car seats where you are leaning back or anything where your knees are higher than your pelvis.

The best way to do this is to spend lots of time kneeling upright, or sitting upright, or on hands and knees. When you sit on a chair, make sure your knees are lower than your pelvis, and your trunk should be tilted slightly forward.

- Watch TV while kneeling on the floor, over a beanbag or cushions, or sit on a dining chair. Try sitting on a dining chair facing (leaning on) the back as well.
- Use yoga positions while resting, reading or watching TV - for example, tailor pose (sitting with your back upright and soles of the feet together, knees out to the sides).
- Sit on a wedge cushion in the car, so that your pelvis is tilted forwards. Keep the seat back upright.
- Don't cross your legs! This reduces the space at the front of the pelvis, and opens it up at the back. For good positioning, the baby needs to have lots of space at the front.
- Don't put your feet up! Lying back with your feet up encourages posterior presentation.
- Sleep on your side, not on your back.
- Avoid deep squatting, which opens up the pelvis and encourages the baby to move down, until you know he/she is the right way round. Jean Sutton recommends squatting on a low stool instead, and keeping your spine upright, not leaning forwards.
- Swimming with your belly downwards is said to be very good for positioning babies - not backstroke, but lots of breaststroke and front crawl. Breaststroke in particular is thought to help with good positioning, because all those leg movements help open your pelvis and settle the baby downwards.
- A Birth Ball can encourage good positioning, both before and during labor.
- Various exercises done on all fours can help, for example wiggling your hips from side to side, or arching your back like a cat, followed by dropping the spine down.

## If your baby is already posterior...

When your baby is in a posterior position, you can try to stop him/her from descending lower. You want to avoid the baby engaging in the pelvis in this position, while you work on encouraging him to turn around. Most babies take a couple of days to turn around when the mother is working hard on positioning.

### *Avoid deep squatting*
- Use the 'knee to chest' position. When on hands and knees, stick your bottom (butt) in the air, to tip the baby back up out of your pelvis so that there is more room for him to turn around.
- Sway your hips while on hands and knees.
- Crawl around on hands and knees. A token 5 minutes on hands and knees is unlikely to do the trick - you need to keep working at this until your baby turns. Try crawling around the carpet for half an hour - while watching TV or listening to music. It is good exercise as well as good for the baby's position!
- Don't put your feet up! Lying back with your feet up encourages posterior presentation.
- Swim belly-down, but avoid kicking with breaststroke legs as this movement is said to encourage the baby to descend in the pelvis [3]. You can still swim breaststroke, but simply kick with straight legs instead of "frogs' legs".

When your baby turns to an anterior position, you can encourage him to descend further into the pelvis - by walking around upright, massaging your bump downwards, deep squatting, and swimming - and now you can use lots of breaststroke "frogs' legs" kicking.

### If your baby is posterior when you go into labor:
These movements can help the baby wriggle through your pelvis, past the ischial spines inside it, by altering the level of your hips. They are also helpful if the baby is anterior but has a presentation problem, for example, his head is tipped to one side.
- In early labor, walk up stairs - sideways if you need to.
- Rock from side to side
- March or 'tread' on the spot
- Step on and off a small stool
- Climb in and out of a birth pool
- The positions listed below may also help.

### For the second stage:
- Use kneeling or all fours positions. Kneeling on one knee can help.
- Supported squatting in second stage, but the mother must be lifted quite high up; her bottom should be at least 45cm (18 inches) off the floor.
- Birth stool seats should be at least 45cm (18 inches) from the floor.
- Avoid lying on your back, semi-reclining, sitting or semi-sitting. These positions all reduce the available space for the baby to turn. Lying on the side is OK.

## Is there any proof that this works?

Midwives and mothers who have learned about, and used, Optimal Fetal Positioning techniques are convinced that it works. There is a wealth of anecdotal evidence in favor of it. However, there have not been any trials or studies on the subject so far, because they would be extremely difficult to organize. Practicing techniques to turn a posterior baby can take a lot of commitment on the part of the mother, which could not be assumed in a randomized trial. There would also be ethical problems with a trial - would mothers in the control group be told not to adopt upright or forward-leaning postures? Or would they simply not be told that taking care with their posture could lead to an easier labor?

There has been one small study which looked at the short-term effects of mothers adopting a hands-and-knees position, compared to sitting, when their baby was in a lateral or posterior position. Mothers were asked to go on hands and knees, or to sit, for a short period of time, and the position of the baby was noted ten minutes afterwards. The study found that babies were far less likely to remain posterior after mothers had been on hands and knees.

However, since the babies' positions were only assessed for ten minutes after one session on hands and knees, this study doesn't tell us very much about the longer-term effects of alterations in the mother's posture. You can read the abstract in the Cochrane Pregnancy and Childbirth Database.

Some good evidence for the effectiveness of the theory comes from its author's own practice. When Jean Sutton was appointed Principal Nurse Midwife at a maternity unit in New Zealand, she emphasized antenatal education on fetal positioning. The transfer rate from maternity unit to hospital fell from 30% to 5 % and the forceps delivery rate fell from 3-4 per month, to 2-4 per year, over a period of several years.

If your baby appears to be in a posterior position, you will probably need to put considerable effort into persuading him to move around. It is no use spending five minutes on your hands and knees every now and then, and then saying "I tried to turn him, but it didn't work".

Optimum Fetal Positioning should be a lifestyle for you, for those last few weeks of pregnancy, not just an occasional distraction. Adopting a 'good' position now and then will not make much difference if you are in 'bad' positions for the majority of the time. A 'good' position is not a magic cure, a pill that you can take to turn your baby. The only person who can get your baby into a good position is you, and unfortunately, you are going to have to do the work to make it happen!

It may be that your baby is going to stay 'sunnyside up' and will just refuse to turn; perhaps that's the way he/she needs to be. However, it can't hurt to try to get the baby to turn. If you do end up having a posterior labor (and they're not all dreadful, but many are harder than they would otherwise be), at least you'll know you did all you could to make things easier for you and your baby.

Reprinted with kind permission of Angela Horn. For more of Angela's work contact www.homebirth.org.uk. Jean Sutton and Pauline Scott, New Zealand, Birth Concepts, 'Understanding and Teaching Optimal Foetal Positioning' Available online from www.nctsales.co.uk.

## What You Need To Know Before You Have Your Baby: Drugs in Pregnancy and Labor - What Effects Will They Have Twenty Years Hence?

Childbirth is a normal physiological event for the majority of women and babies. As a species we have been spectacularly successful. However, since near universal hospitalization, for the majority of women in developed countries, childbirth has become a medical event, where pregnancy and labor are processed, monitored and controlled by the protocols and policies of the medical profession from beginning to end. This came about through a system of childbirth care which was planned and controlled by medical experts. Childbirth was not considered a medical event and doctors were only involved when childbirth became complicated. Over the centuries, and with the urbanization of the population, which enabled doctors to establish lying-in hospitals and thereby have a captive group of women on whom they could carry out research, the medical profession became more interested in controlling childbirth. This can be best achieved by having large, centralized, maternity units.

Although many women understand the benefits of a normal birth and see pregnancy and birth as a normal process, few women giving birth in large centralized medical establishments will experience a normal birth and many will find themselves and their babies subjected to a whole range of powerful drugs and medical procedures. Women, allegedly, give informed consent for their use. The reality, however, is that the majority of women have little information about drugs in labor. Drugs are often offered by the staff as a replacement for good support from a midwife who should be with the woman throughout her labour and be able to counteract the fear or anxiety she may feel as a result of being in an alien/hospital environment surrounded by strangers and where she has little real control.

The propaganda promotes the "advantages" of drug use, but little is said about the disadvantages. Particularly the long-term effects and it is those effects that are addressed in this article.

**Thalidomide** All drugs have unwanted effects, some more serious than others. In the 1950s and 60s thousands of babies, all over the world, were born with severe limb abnormalities; as a direct result of their mothers having been prescribed thalidomide, to reduce nausea, during their pregnancies. It took ten years for researchers to establish that thalidomide was to blame; despite the children suffering gross abnormalities of their limbs. Meanwhile, the medical profession, and the drug companies, vigorously denied any connection. How long would it have taken had the abnormalities been subtle?

Now, however, there is a suspicion - disputed by some doctors - that thalidomide has reached a second generation (Driscoll M, 1995) Of 386 babies born to the original thalidomide damaged children, eight are malformed with deformities which are suspiciously similar to the deformities suffered by their parents. Some doctors argue that the parents had been wrongly diagnosed as suffering from a thalidomide induced abnormality; they suggest the parents had a misdiagnosed congenital abnormality which the children have now inherited.

**Diethylstilboestrol (DES)** During the 1940s and 50s the drug diethylstilboestrol was given to pregnant women in the belief that it could prevent miscarriage. Unfortunately, it was widely adopted, particularly in the United States, before any randomized clinical trial was conducted to show whether it was effective. When such a trial was eventually done the drug was shown not to work. Nonetheless, some doctors continued to use it. The time bomb effect came to light in 1971 with the publication of a paper which revealed that a cluster of young women in one town had developed an unusual form of cancer - clear cell carcinoma of the vagina (Herbst, 1971). Had they developed a more common cancer (squamous cell cancer of the cervix) it would have been much less likely that the link would have been made. These women also had other problems, such as abnormalities of the genital tract, some of which have led to problems giving birth. However, more subtle long-term effects were only discovered when British researchers (Vassey et al, 1983) studied the now grown-up offspring of women who had been involved in a randomized clinical trial (half had been given diethylstilboestrol when pregnant, the other half were controls and, therefore, were not given it) and found that psychiatric disease (especially depression and anxiety) was about twice that of those who had not taken the drug.

Further studies have shown that 40% to 50% of DES exposed daughters have pronounced uterine structural abnormalities; and increased risks for ectopic pregnancy, miscarriage and premature birth. Infertility has also been reported in the exposed daughters (Senekjian, 1988) and diminished fertility in the sons (Stillman, 1982)

More than four to eight times as many of the DES exposed children went on to have tubal pregnancies than the unexposed. A quarter of all pregnancies among the DES exposed children went on to miscarry compared with the normal 10% rate. Premature birth occurred in three times as many babies (15% of the DES exposed as those of the non-exposed) (Appleford, 1994).

For DES exposed sons, adverse effects included testicular abnormalities, undescended testes, sperm abnormalities and low sperm counts. (Stillman, 1982) Exposed children were significantly more likely to have serious mental illness and boys were less likely to have married.

We suggest that many of the non physical, but serious adverse effects, would not have been identified but for the fact that exposed girls had developed a particularly unusual cancer.

In the USA the grand-daughters of women given stilboestrol in pregnancy are now suing for injuries they suffered because of alleged stilboestrol-induced abnormalities in the genital tracts of their mothers who were exposed in the womb. This is an example of how damage may be transmitted from generation to generation. One would have expected, therefore, that the medical profession would be particularly careful about using drugs in pregnancy and labour.

**Pethidine (Demerol)** One of the most common drugs used in the labour ward is pethidine. It is a synthetic, addictive, narcotic drug which is similar to Morphine. It is also known as Meperidine and, in America, Demerol. It has become the drug of first choice for the majority of midwives, mainly because it is the only pharmacological narcotic which midwives are licensed to prescribe. Women often find it very difficult indeed to cope with the increased pain caused by drug induced or accelerated labours and, commonly, they will be given a dose of 150mg of pethidine, yet those midwives who use pethidine sparingly often give a much smaller dose (e.g. 25mg) and claim it is just as effective.

Researchers from Stockholm, however, found that pethidine did not relieve labour pain and commented that "it seems unethical and medically incorrect to meet the request for analgesia by giving her heavy sedation." (Olofsson et al, 1996)

It has been suggested that if pethidine came into the market now it would be rejected as a form of pain relief in labour because of its high rate of ineffectiveness and its serious adverse effects.

## Adverse effects in babies

An intramuscular injection of pethidine acts on the mother within 20 minutes and readily crosses the placenta. The baby has greater sensitivity to the drug than an adult, because of the immaturity of the blood-brain barrier and the circulatory bypass of the liver (Burt, 1971). Before the birth the mother's liver processes the drug, but if any of the drug remains the baby's immature liver has to take over this processing once the baby is born.

Most midwives try to ensure that pethidine is not given if the baby is expected to be born within an hour, because of the risk that the drug will still be present in the baby's system at birth. However, research shows that pethidine is most likely to cause breathing difficulties if the drug is administered two or three hours before birth. The higher the dose to the mother, the greater the effect on the fetus (Yerby, 1996). As the baby's liver is immature, it takes a great deal longer for the baby to eliminate the drug from its system (usually 18-23 hours) although 95% of the drug is excreted in 2-3 days. This can have significant implications for breast feeding. Babies suffering the effects of pethidine are often drowsy and unresponsive and researchers have demonstrated that 'Pethidine proved to be the (drug) most inhibiting to breast feeding' By breast feeding, the mother, often unknowingly, gives the baby a second dose of pethidine as the drug is transferred to the baby through the breastmilk (Rajan, 1994). She may not be aware that pethidine is the cause of her 'sleepy' baby and her problems getting the baby latched on.

Little research has been done into the long-term effects of pethidine. However, it has been shown that infants with high pethidine exposure were more likely to cry when handled on days 7, 21 and 42, as were those with a high cord blood concentration on day 21. Pethidine also reduced the infant's ability to quiet himself once aroused and this effect can last for up to six weeks (Belsey, 1981). The researchers only investigated this far and it is interesting that researchers consider three to six weeks to be 'long-term', when our definition would be in years.

For those babies whose breathing is depressed naloxone is given to reverse pethidine's effects, but the reversal is only temporary unless it is given in an adult dose (Weiner, 1977). We know of no research which investigates the short or long-term effects of naloxone on the baby.

## Adverse Effects in the Mother

One of the criticisms AIMS' members have consistently made of obstetrically managed births, is that once the woman is deemed to be in labour there is pressure to deliver all babies as quickly as possible; yet there is no research showing a fast birth is of benefit to either the mother or the baby. We know of no study which asked women whether or not they wanted a faster but more painful labour; or of any studies showing that it was beneficial to babies to have a fast labour. Ironically, a study by Thomson and Hillier (1994) showed that women who had pethidine during labour had labours which lasted four hours longer than women who did not have this drug.

It is extremely difficult to assess the level of pain a woman is experiencing because different women react to pain in different ways. Interestingly, when a woman does not experience pain relief from pethidine, or other drugs, she will often be told that she has a 'low pain threshold'. The problem is attributed to women rather than seen as a failure of the drug to act effectively, despite the fact that pethidine is known to be an ineffective form of pain relief. In a survey of pain relief in childbirth (Chamberlain, 1993) 84% of midwives rated pethidine as very good or good, compared with only 71% of women and 72% of partners. The authors speculated that: "perhaps the drowsiness of the woman following the administration of pethidine is associated with effective pain relief by the midwife?" From the woman's perspective, pethidine has been described as causing a loss of control, disorientation, and dizziness and as one mother described it: "I felt that my brain had gone out to lunch. I could not put a sentence together, but it did nothing for the pain - it just shut me up".

Women who end up with caesarean sections have often experienced induced and accelerated labours; because this type of labour is more painful, women usually need pharmacological pain relief. Pethidine will be one of the drugs they are most likely to have been given during their labour. However, pethidine delays maternal gastric emptying and, together with sedation, increases the risk of aspiration (breathing in the stomach's contents) and thus the danger to the woman of general anaesthetic if a caesarean operation is advised (Olofsson, 1997).

Chamberlain's Study Pain and its Relief in Childbirth (1993) found that for the woman, pethidine came bottom of the list in terms of adequate pain relief, satisfaction with labour, and feeling in control of labour and birth and being in good physical and mental health afterwards. Women who had been given pethidine were least likely to want to use it in future births.

## Epidural Anaesthesia

The latest research paper (revealing the inadequacy of pethidine's pain relieving effects) instead of urging non-pharmacological methods of pain relief (for example, the wider use of water pools) suggests that epidural anaesthesia should now be widely available (Olofsson, 1996). Evidently, there are few professionals who are worried about the adverse effects of this drug.

Researchers in the UK (Rosenblatt et al, 1981) published a six-week follow-up of the effects of epidural anaesthesia, which showed that immediately after birth, infants with greater exposure to bupivacaine (the drug used in epidurals) in utero were most likely to be cyanotic (suffering from a lack of oxygen) and unresponsive to their surroundings. Visual skills and alertness decreased significantly particularly on the first day of life, but also throughout the next six weeks; these effects increased with greater amounts of the drug found in the baby's blood,. Adverse effects of bupivacaine levels on the infant's motor organization, his ability to control his own state of consciousness and his physiological response to stress were also observed. Interestingly, this study considered six-week to be a "long-term", but we need to know what the long-term effects are at five, ten, twenty or fifty years? Before consenting to an epidural every woman should watch Lennard Righard's video which shows the startling difference in the behavior of babies who have been exposed to epidurals compared with those who have not. The video was filmed to demonstrate how babies, when left to themselves, can wriggle up to latch onto the mother's breast. The video shows how the epidural exposed babies lie like beached whales on their mothers' bellies and are actually incapable of making the vigorous movements which were noticed in the undrugged babies.

Women who choose water for pain relief have been warned that a rise in the water temperature over 37C could cause a rise in the mother's temperature and theoretically result in brain damage in the baby. There has been no research to support this suggestion. As a result, however, many UK hospitals have restricted access to water pools, although there has not been a single recorded case of such damage. However, research by Lieberman (1997) revealed that intrapartum (during labour and birth) fever greater than 100.4F occurred in 14.5% of women receiving an epidural, and if these labours lasted longer than 18 hours the fever rates increased to 36%. As far as we are aware, not a single paediatrician has expressed concern about this risk. It is not always obvious to the distressed mothers that the unpleasant blood tests, lumbar punctures etc., that their newborns might have to endure in the Special Care Baby Unit (to rule out the possibility of an infection) or that their prolonged stay in the hospital was brought about because of their epidural induced fever in labour.

## Brain development

Some parts of the brain are fairly well developed at the time a human being is born, but other parts are not. Some of them, particularly the cerebellum, are very under-developed, and the introduction of toxic substances during this period of rapid development, even for a single dose (it doesn't have to be a repeated administration) can either kill cells or cause alterations in the cells that are present. Cells proliferate in the cerebellum - and then migrate into their final position and link up with other cells. Both the rate of cell death and the patterns of migration of cells in the cerebellum have been shown to be very sensitive to the introduction of toxic substances (Brackbill Y, 1979).

In the human being, the period of vulnerability to central nervous system damage from exposure to drugs and chemicals lasts a long time. Even after birth, important areas of the brain are still developing and differentiating rapidly, because of this rapid period of growth they are most vulnerable to damage and at highest risk. It has been estimated for example that the brain growth spurt in the cerebellum (the hind brain, situated above the area where the spine joins the cranium) lasts for eighteen months after birth and in the hippocampus, for about four and a half years.

Yvonne Brackbill in her submission to the Food and Drugs Authority commented that at that time there had been at least 40 studies of neuro-behavioural changes in human infants that were observed after administration of anaesthetic and pre-anaesthetic agents to their mothers during labour and delivery. "None has shown that drugs enhance or improve behavioural functioning in infants" (Brackbill Y, 1979).

While the process of cell migration is not yet fully understood, present knowledge of neurobiology suggests that the normal biochemical message left along the pathway of the neuron by the preceding cell (as it travels to its proper place within the central nervous system) leaves a biochemical message along the pathway which directs the next brain cell into place.

Drug-induced biochemical alterations within the brain of the about-to-be born or new-born infant have the potential for permanently disrupting the normal link-up of the baby's brain cells by altering the biochemical markers which guide the cells into their proper places. It is somewhat similar to the unintentional spilling of a chemical over telephone wires which are being connected according to the colour code at the end of each wire. The chemical removes the colour from the wire ends. The technician must continue to connect the wires, not knowing exactly which wires to connect with which. The circuitry is completed: it functions, but imperfectly.

Desmond Bardon, (1984) a respected British psychiatrist, asked what prolonged exposure to the drugs given to a mother in labour might mean to the later neurologic development and behaviour of the offspring? Could it be that dyslexia is one of the results?

## Drug addiction

When a baby is born to an undrugged mother and not whisked away to be washed, wrapped, and weighed, the baby will look around, respond to its mother's voice and seek her breast. If the mother and baby are not disturbed they will respond to each other and start the process of "bonding". Women who have drugs in labour are often unaware that the major reason their baby is unresponsive is because it is affected by the drugs which the mother had during the labour, and if the lights in the room are bright it will have its eyes tightly closed.

The effects of these drugs are not just their capacity to interfere with breast feeding or sleepy babies in the short term. In the developed world there is an epidemic of behavioural problems, dyslexia and drug addiction. I suggest that one of the reasons for this - amongst others - is the over-use of powerful drugs in labour.

In the United States it appears that women who smoke or drink alcohol in pregnancy can be publicly chastised. If they take heroin, or other street drugs, they can find themselves in jail or threatened with removal of the baby after the birth and even their other children as well. It is surprising, therefore, that so few people seem to be concerned about the powerful addictive drugs which are commonly used on the labour ward, and few appear even concerned enough to research the effects these drugs can have on the still-developing fetal brain and other long-term effects on women and babies.

There are plenty of studies examining the immediate effects of drugs in labour, but where are the studies examining the long-term effects, which can emerge, five, ten, twenty or even fifty years later.

We are a drug-centered society. The majority of the population uses prescribed drugs and a growing proportion also use illegal drugs. We could be sitting on a time bomb if we persist in ignoring the research because of the disturbing implications. No one wants to admit that accepted practices might be creating drug addicts, for example; but that is what many childbirth activists, and some doctors and midwives, believe the overuse of drugs in pregnancy and childbirth is achieving.

In a well designed case control led study at the Karolinska Institute in Stockholm researchers compared children exposed to pain relieving drugs in labour, with those who were not, and discovered an increased risk of drug addiction later in life (Jacobson B et al, 1990). In 1988 they showed that when a large dose of nitrous oxide was given to the mother the child was five and a half times more likely to become an amphetamine addict than a brother or sister born to the same parents (Jacobson B et al, 1988). In a more recent paper in the British Medical Journal they compared patients who had died from opiate addiction with brothers and sisters and found that if the mothers had had opiates or barbiturates or larger doses of nitrous oxide the risk of opiate addiction to the child in later life was increased by 4.7 times (Jacobson B et al, 1990). In a further study they discovered that the risk of drug addiction was related to the hospital in which the baby was born. In other words, the likelihood of a child becoming drug addicted in later life depended on the labour ward policies of the hospital his mother chose for the birth: "For the amphetamine addicts, hospital birth was found to be an important risk factor even after controlling for residential area" (Nyberg K et al, 1993). Jacobson and Nyberg's research suggests that the use of opiates, barbiturates and nitrous oxide in labour causes imprinting in the babies, and we are now seeing the effects of this.

The US Department of Health and Human Services estimated that one out of every 9 American children is significantly learning disabled despite having normal intelligence. Seventy five percent of these children are born at full term into middle and upper class families. The National Institutes of Health, in the USA, estimate that 75% to 85% of all disabled children in the US were born within the normal range of birth weight and gestational age and had no familial or sociologic predisposing factors. (Haire, 1989)

Desmond Bardon suggested that a significant proportion of the millions of children and youths in the USA who are afflicted with significant mental and neurologic dysfunction are the victims of obstetric medications administered with the very best of intentions to the mother during labour and birth in medicalized maternity units (Bardon, 1984). Not only have his concerns not been addressed, but since that time even more women and babies have been, and continue to be, subjected to high levels of drugs in labour. Little has been done to investigate the possibility that the huge increases in drug addiction and associated crime are a direct result of the drugs used on the labour wards. As Association for Improvements in Maternity Services frequently points out, while various agencies work hard to pull the bodies out of the river, no one is investigating who might be pushing them in upstream. It is time they did."

Reprinted with kind permission from Beverley A Lawrence Beech, Hon Chair - AIMS and Midwifery Today. Issue 50, Summer 1999, www.midwiferytoday.com. Beverley A. Lawrence Beech is a researcher, writer and speaker. She is honorary chair of the Association for Improvements in the Maternity Services, (AIMS), and can be contacted through www.aims.org.uk. Midwifery Today is a magazine and an E-magazine that contains top childbirth research from around the world. Additional articles on any topic regarding childbirth can be found at www.midwiferytoday.com.

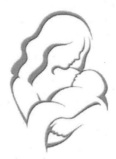

# Chapter Seven - Seventh Month

This is a good time to preview the section in this book on newborn care. Visualize what you will do with your baby on your first day together. More women are using Kangaroo Care on the first day, letting baby sleep or nap on your chest with skin to skin contact after feeding to help maintain the close connection your baby felt to you in your womb. It is a wonderful way to soothe both mother and baby in the first days together.     Kangaroo     care by both partners creates deeper bonding and attachment with your baby. The scent of your baby actually releases certain hormones to help both partners bond more closely with the baby. This is why we can't resist kissing baby's sweet cheeks. Their scent is truly irresistible.

To relieve pressure on your body while sleeping add a second pillow to prop you up as you sleep. This can help you to breathe easier and can help relieve heartburn. Sleeping with a pillow tucked slightly under your belly can also relieve any muscle straining you may be feeling. Body pillows give great support to your expanding body and belly.

Stock up on sodium-free club soda. Club soda has no calories and is great for quenching your thirst. Keep a stock in your car and at work.

Purchase good slippers with some elastic support.

Increase your outdoor activities. Animals give birth faster and easier when they are let free once a day rather than being penned up. A rancher did an independent study by putting half his pregnant cattle within the corral day and night, the other half were led to a feeding area a distance away every evening. Twice as many complications arose in the cows that had been penned up. Giving birth is a tremendous physical challenge to your body and the stronger you become physically, the easier the challenge.

Walking will ease lower back pain and is a great way to unwind from the day. If you have back pain you may want to walk on a treadmill at a gym or walk on grass. Shopping malls have tile placed upon concrete which can create additional pressure on your back and legs. You will also find that walking strengthens muscles you will be using during your labor and delivery. Stronger legs allow you to maintain an assisted squatting position for a longer period of time. A squatting position is one of the best and most natural positions for birth, making for an easier delivery for both mother and baby.

Can't sleep near the end of your pregnancy? Get up and do something useful or relaxing. Nature is getting you ready for the time when you will have to get up in the middle of the night, so learn to use the time for your benefit. There may be many nights when your baby is a few months old and she is awake at 2:00 a.m. for one or two hours.

## Kegels for Pregnancy and Childbirth

Kegels reduce urinary incontinence, help relieve and reduce hemorrhoids, help you to create a faster and easier delivery and will get you ready and toned again to resume a good sex life. To locate your pelvic muscle and do the Kegel exercises; when urinating start and stop the flow of urine, this will isolate the target muscle area which is the PC muscle. Tighten these muscles and hold to the count of ten, then release and tighten again.

Latest research shows that holding your PC muscles for a long rather than a short period of time will condition these muscles more quickly. Count to ten and slowly release for the greatest effect in the shortest amount of time. To keep your PC muscle toned it is important to practice Kegel exercises on a daily basis, both before and after the birth. Do sets of ten or twenty throughout the day.

Other variations include; Slow Kegels: tighten the PC muscle as if to stop the urine. Hold for a slow count of three, and then relax. Repeat ten times. Quick Kegels: Tighten and relax the PC muscle as quickly as you can, five times. Relax and repeat ten times. Pull in-Push Out Kegels: Pull up the entire pelvic floor as though trying to suck water into the vagina. Then push out or bear down as if trying to push imaginary water out. This exercise uses the stomach abdominal muscles as well as the PC muscle. Do this four or five times in a row. Repeat ten times.

## Sex after Childbirth

Pregnancy, labor and delivery are taxing on a woman's body. How the mother cares for herself and is cared for, after the baby comes, depends on the nature of the delivery and whether there have been any complications. It is important to get up and around as soon as possible after childbirth for the healing of your body. Be guided by your own body.

Activities such as work, sex, housework, and exercise should be resumed only when you feel ready. In Western culture, people have demanding schedules and want instant results. It is therefore important for a woman to be aware of the stress her body has endured and the recovery it must make. Sleep deprivation, breastfeeding, and caring for your infant and yourself make extra demands on your body. Pacing yourself and taking slow steps are key in maintaining normal activities and optimum health.

Good nutrition while breastfeeding remains as important now as during pregnancy. Eating a varied diet with plenty of whole foods and fluids still applies. Aggressive dieting during this time of healing and nurturing is detrimental to the health of both mother and baby.

A woman must determine for herself when she is ready to resume intercourse. Probably the most important thing to feed a healthy sex life is a healthy relationship. Parents are often taught that children come first. But if a marriage or relationship is not attended to; there is no family. Partners should get out by themselves on a regular basis and find ways to attend to each other emotionally and not just sexually. In this way you will reconnect with the relationship you had before your first baby.

Setting aside ten or fifteen minutes per day for discussing the events of the day is a pleasant way for partners to reconnect. Sleep is a powerful aphrodisiac and can contribute to both partners enjoyment of sex when you set the alarm for the middle of the night. Hiring a baby-sitter away from home in the middle of the day when both partners are more rested can also help you to resume sexual activity and intimacy. Doing Kegel exercises throughout your pregnancy and after birth will quickly recondition your body. Using extra lubricant during lovemaking at this time can also make sexual activity more enjoyable.

Fear of another pregnancy often decreases a woman's sexual desires after childbirth. Plan ahead for your birth control method. While breastfeeding appears to suppress ovulation somewhat and helps in the spacing of children, it is not a guaranteed form of birth control. The baby's frequent sucking while breastfeeding initiates the release of hormones that appear to suspend menstruation and ovulation. However, it is possible to ovulate and become fertile before menstruation returns.

There are several effective, safe and inexpensive forms of birth control that can be used, for example, natural family planning which involves the daily charting of fertility signs, such as basal body temperature, consistency of the cervical mucus, as well as the newest hand-held microscopes that show you visually, using your saliva, your personal ovulation cycle. Do not use oral contraceptives while breastfeeding.

## Planning for a Homebirth

Excerpted from Informed Home Birth Magazine by Rahima Baldwin Dancy, founder of the Informed Homebirth and the Informed Birth & Parenting Association.

"Some people feel that women selfishly choose homebirth by putting their own experience above the safety of the baby. This is simply not true; everyone wants a healthy mother and a healthy baby. Couples who have their baby at home know that statistics bear out the safety of assisted homebirth for low-risk mothers; they also recognize that there are many advantages for the baby as well as the mother and the entire family.

Advantages for the baby include that she or he is more likely to be born vaginally, without the breathing difficulties often caused by cesarean birth or anesthesia. There is less likelihood of infection when the baby is with the mother than in the newborn nursery. The baby's experience at birth can be recognized and made as gentle as possible. Routine procedures such as deep suctioning, suctioning the stomach, scrubbing the baby, vitamin K shots, eye ointments and the like can be avoided.

Advantages for the mother include not being subjected to routine procedures such as electronic monitoring, IVs, shave, prep, enema or stirrups. She can eat and walk freely, her body working with nature. She will have continuity of care with the same attendants, increasing her safety. She is more likely to be treated and her progress evaluated as an individual, rather than being sacrificed to protocols or averages. She is much less likely to need pain killing drugs, forceps or a cesarean section when she has attendants who feel that birth is a normal physical function. She is comfortable in her own surroundings, relaxed and able to labor and deliver in the same place. She has less chance of infection and episiotomy. Postpartum depression is more uncommon since there are no unnecessary interventions or separation.

Advantages for the family include husbands in their own home rather than someone allowing them to be present. They can participate as fully as they want. Other children can be present as appropriate. A homebirth becomes an integral part of family life, helping to ease postpartum adjustment for all members of the family."

## Pregnancy & Massage Therapy

"Massage, the art of therapeutic bodywork, has been practiced from time immemorial by both ancient and primitive peoples. Concepts which linked the body to the mind and spirit were once discounted as "unscientific" in the west, and the human body came to be regarded as a sophisticated machine. Yet in the light of the development of modern psychology and a more sophisticated knowledge of anatomy and physiology, health care professionals are beginning to reexamine touch therapy. As we confront the challenge of understanding how personal growth, character, physical structure, and health and disease relate to one another, we begin to create a new matrix -- "the bodymind".* * Term coined by Ken Dychtwald in his book Bodymind.

Bodymind is the concept that health and disease don't just happen to us; they are active processes reflecting psychological and somatic harmony. As more is learned in research on the brain, the connection between mind and illness becomes understandable. The brain masterminds or indirectly influences every function of the body: blood pressure, heart rate, immune responses and hormones. The old saying "name your poison" applies to the semantics and symbols of disease. People have long spoken of a "broken heart" as the symbol of a disappointing relationship: research now shows a connection between loneliness and heart disease!

Over the years, our bodies become walking autobiographies that tell friends and strangers alike of the minor stresses and strains of our lives. If one has an accident, distortions resulting from injury can become a permanent part of our body pattern. Our musculature reflects old anxieties-fear, depression, bravado, stoicism- locked into our bodies as patterns in our sensory-motor systems. Our body's tight patterns begin to contribute to our locked-in mental processes. For instance, just as the body is constricted by the mind's grief, the mind is constricted by the body's stubborn memory of what the mind used to feel.

The sum total of this is that massage has unlimited possibilities for human development from two different angles. On the one hand, based on physiological principles, massage can provide the means to relieve the incredible stress and strain to which we are subjected day after day in modern living. For those to whom pain and stiffness are a habitual way of life, bodywork can provide a means to experience how it feels to have a body that can breathe, stand and move more freely, unconstricted by tight muscles and not drained by energy-consuming tension. On the other hand, there are a diverse array of therapies that deeply massage, manipulate, loosen and change the body's neuromuscular system, its orientation to gravity, and its symmetry.

There is no other time in which bodywork can have as important an application than during pregnancy.

When we begin to visualize pregnancy as far more than a physical state, and see it as a profound emotional, mental and spiritual process, it is clear that massage can be of great benefit to the pregnant mother. Women have long held the amazing ability to influence the state of their bodies with their thoughts and feelings, and conversely, to allow their physical appearance or state of health to dominate how they feel about themselves as individuals. How many of us have created an acne breakout when nervous about a new date, or allowed the "bad hair day" syndrome to taint an otherwise perfectly normal day with irritability and gloom?

During pregnancy and childbearing, the enormous influx of hormones combined with weight gain, altered body shape, and the normal biophysical and structural discomforts caused by increased blood volume and a shifting center of gravity, all contribute to many pregnant women feeling downright uncomfortable, emotionally and physically! Massage can provide an excellent means not only for relieving body stress, but also for helping her deal with emotional fears and concerns. When a woman feels integrated and healthy in her body and mind, she will manifest a more positive birth experience.

How is it possible that simply "rubbing" the skin can presume to live up to claims of being one of the most effective means to influence the structures and functions of body and mind? The skin is the largest sensory organ of the human body, arising in the human embryo from the same cell layers as the nervous system, the ectoderm. Ashley Montague writes in Touching:

> The surface area of the skin has an enormous number of sensory receptors receiving stimuli of heat, cold, touch, pressure, and pain. A piece of skin the size of a quarter contains more than 3 million cells, 100-340 sweat glands, 50 nerve endings and three feet of blood vessels. It is estimated that there are some 50 receptors/100 sq. mm., a total of 640,000 sensory receptors. The number of sensory fibers from the skin entering the spinal cord is well over half a million.

In a sense, the nervous system is part of the skin, or the skin is an external nervous system, conveying knowledge of the environment to the organism. In the evolution of the senses, the tactile system was the first system to come into being in all species. The sense most closely associated with the skin, the sense of touch, is the earliest to develop in the human embryo.

Touch means contact, a relationship with what lies outside our own periphery. For humans touch is of vital importance, giving reassurance, warmth, pleasure and vitality. It tells us that we are not alone. As infants, it is primarily through touch that we explore and make sense of the world; the loving touch of our parents is essential to our growth. The cuddling and stroking we receive in infancy helps us build a healthy image of ourselves and nurtures the feeling that we are accepted and loved.

Psychologists have demonstrated that our perception of how much we are touched relates to how we value ourselves, our self-esteem. Patients denied skin contact report feeling acutely isolated, cut off from the warmth of human touch- hence the concept of "solitary confinement" as the ultimate punishment. With the increased physiological and emotional stress of pregnancy, an occasional massage can be of significant benefit.

**Some of the primary physical effects of bodywork are:**
1. Massage serves to heighten circulation to the skin by increasing blood flow to the veins and surface capillaries, promoting better cellular nutrition and elimination.
2. Massage increases production of red and white blood cells, especially useful in cases of anemia.
3. The work of the heart is lessened due to improved circulation.
4. Massage stimulates the activity of sweat and oil glands creating more radiant and supple skin.
5. Massage influences blood and lymph vessels by direct mechanical action, putting pressure on the vessel walls which propels the movement of blood, and stimulating the vasomotor nerves which control constriction and relaxation of blood vessels and determine the amount of blood reaching the area being massaged.
6. Massage acts as a mechanical cleanser, pushing along lymph and hastening the elimination of wastes and toxic debris.
7. Massage relaxes muscle spasms, improves muscle tone and elasticity, and helps prevent atrophy resulting from inactivity.

8. Muscle tissue, tired by work or exercise, is restored more quickly as waste products of fatigue (i.e. lactic acid) are readily removed, and replacement nutrients replenished by increased circulation.
9. Massage stretches connective tissue, and improves its circulation and nutrition, reducing the danger of fibrosis and preventing the formation of adhesions.
10. Massage improves circulation and nutrition to joints.

**Some of the psychological effects of bodywork are:**
1. Massage helps relieve muscle tension and corresponding mental tension.
2. Deep tissue massage helps free up fascia (connective tissue) and muscles, allowing the body to assume a more integrated posture.
3. By releasing chronically held trauma and reconnecting the natural flow and balance of the organism, touch therapy encourages growth and openness on all levels of functioning.
4. Gentle stoking has a sedative affect on the nervous system, promoting deep relaxation.
5. Allowing the intimacy of touch creates a state of trust and receptivity which facilitates clearer mental and emotional perception.
6. Massage can assist the integration of emotional, mental or spiritual transformation on a cellular level.
7. The sense of renewed health and vitality experienced following a bodywork session improves self esteem and consequently esteem for others.

Clearly then, massage is particularly beneficial for expectant mothers as it not only promotes physical well being, but also helps prepare women psychologically and spiritually for the process of labor and birth. Although a professional massage may be a wonderful way to experience bodywork, it is by no means the only way. During pregnancy, friends or partners can experiment with different strokes and pressures to help relieve some of the natural stress and tensions of the expectant mother. There are many excellent books giving basic instruction in technique for the novice. The key is to remain sensitive at all times to her needs, and to allow her to communicate where and how she is comfortable being touched. Be creative, open and loving.

Reprinted with kind permission of Shelly Girard, B.S., M.P.H., L.M., C.P.M.,C.M.T. Shelly Girard is a Certified Massage Therapist, Licensed

Midwife, and Certified Professional Midwife with 28 years experience in body/mind medicine. She received her Master's in Public Health from the University of California Los Angeles in June, 2000. For further information contact www.socalbirth.org

## Shopping Tips

This is a good time to being assembling your layette. You can cut the cost of your layette in half by purchasing many of the items your baby will need second hand. Most infant clothing is only worn a few months and can easily go through a number of babies. Go to garage sales. Ask friends and family for items they no longer have use for. Look for second hand and consignment stores in your city for good quality clothing at excellent prices. To get the best value for your money buy most of your baby's clothing after your baby arrives. It is easy to buy too much in the wrong sizes.

If you find a mother to purchase clothing and baby accessories from stay in touch with her and call her two or three times a year to see if she has anything else she would like to sell. Talk to other mothers about what they found to be invaluable to have for the baby and what things they really didn't need. Purchase your crib and car seat new or nearly new. These two products are continually updated each year to provide our babies with the best in safety. Support the manufacturers in updating these products by buying your crib and car seat new, your newborn deserves the best in these two safety products.

Sample Layette Purchase
- 1 Dozen One Piece Undershirts
- 1 Dozen One Piece Jumpers
- 6 Large Flannel Receiving Blankets
- 4 Booties/Socks
- 1 Sweater/Hat
- 1 Snow Suit or Coat
- 2 Crib Sheets/2 Waterproof Pads/1 Bumper Pad
- 1 Quilt/Bassinet mattress and bedding
- 6 Washcloths
- Baby Soap
- Baby Body Wash
- Baby Brush and Comb
- Q-Tips for Umbilical Cord Care only. Never use Q-tips in your baby's ear as you can easily puncture the ear drum or push accumulated wax even

further into the ear canal. Use a drop or two of mineral oil and a small piece of cotton to gently remove excess wax from the outside of the ear.

- Saline Solution for Umbilical Cord Care
- Thermometer – Digital ear thermometers or underarm thermometers are best.
- Baby Nail File and Clippers
- Sponge Bath Rest
- Diaper Pail
- 4 Dozen Prefolded Cloth Diapers
- Size One Disposable Diapers for Traveling – Newborn size is often too small.
- 4 Pair Breathable Nylon Waterproof Pants with Velcro attachments.
- Hot/Cold Gel Packs for Breast Engorgement

**Your layette for the first year may also include:**
Crib & Mattress, (not necessary at once if you use a family bed or bassinet), Change Table, Chest of Drawers, Infant Car Seat, Carriage or Stroller, High Chair, Safety Gate, Baby Swing, Rocking Chair, Sling, Breastfeeding Pillow, and assorted toys and books.

You can reduce your costs by shopping smart, breastfeeding instead of bottle-feeding, and using cloth diapers instead of disposables. If you are unsure of whether you prefer cloth or disposable diapers, hire a diaper service for the first two months. As a new client you can usually ask for two weeks free.

A diaper service with pick-up and drop-off once a week, is convenient, hassle-free, ecological and an excellent service for any mother. Today's pre-folded cloth diapers are quickly and easily changed with Velcro strips instead of pins and breathable outer nylon covers instead of plastic pants. Cloth diapers are kinder on your baby's bottom and on the environment. Many mothers are using both cloth and disposable diapers. A diaper service also saves you from that mad dash to the store for something you will need everyday for the first two years.

Cloth diapers reduce the number and types of rashes your baby may have from using disposable diapers and they can save you money from buying expensive prescription creams. Adding Borax to the wash cycle will help to keep the cloth diapers odor free and sanitized. When laundering your cloth diapers dissolve Borax into the water before adding diapers and then allow them to soak. This will change the acidic nature of the diaper to an alkaline nature. You may find it convenient to use both cloth and alternative disposable diapers. You can now purchase chemical-free disposable cotton diapers.

Undershirts with attached bottoms are an excellent buy and most will last through three months of growing. You will find this to be the best uniform for your baby as they absorb leakage and keep your baby warm all over. These undershirts and flannel receiving blankets make the best baby uniform; having an abundance of both on hand makes it easier to clean up burps and spills.

## What You Need To Know Before You Have Your Baby: The Best Care for a Premature Baby

"Kangaroo Care, a program of skin-to-skin contact between parent and child, is part of the revolution in the care of premature infants. First researched in Latin America, Kangaroo Care was tested around the world during the 1980's and it is quickly becoming a popular treatment for premature infants. Neonatologists are seeing great improvements in newborns who participate in Kangaroo Care. Not only do the sleeping and breathing patterns of premature infants improve, the babies appear to relax and become content from the touch of their parents' skin. Parents also benefit psychologically because they are allowed to play an active rather than a passive role in the recovery of their infant.

Scores of international scientific studies have shown that Kangaroo Care offers the preterm infant many physical and emotional benefits. These benefits include:
- A more stable heart rate.
- More regular breathing.
- Improved dispersion of oxygen throughout the body.
- Prevention of cold stress.
- Longer periods of sleep during which the brain matures.
- More rapid weight gain.
- Reduction of purposeless activity which simply burns calories at the expense of the infant's growth and health.
- Decreased crying.
- Longer periods of alertness.
- Opportunities to breastfeed.
- Greater opportunities for both parents and infant to attach.
- Increased likelihood of being discharged from the hospital sooner.

The benefits to parents have also been well documented. Those who have practiced Kangaroo Care feel more positive about the birth experience despite its inherent difficulty. They are eager and ready to bring their babies home and feel confident in handling them because they have already enjoyed opportunities to create a loving relationship. This is true of fathers as well as mothers. In short, Kangaroo Care helps premature babies to recover as it enables their parents to lovingly, actively, and positively participate in their care.

## Easy Steps for Kangaroo Care

Get yourself ready by having a meal and emptying your bladder as you'll be sitting for a one or two hour period. If you have a cold or the flu postpone the session until you're absolutely well, unless you are in a private room or at home. Your baby will be protected but the others may not. Make sure you are well away from any drafts or hot sunny windows. A large chair with arm rests and a foot rest will give you the best support. Use a telephone book, boxes, stool or whatever else is at hand. If the chair is not equipped with a foot rest elevate your legs to half the height of the chair to ensure good circulation in your legs.

Your infant must not be totally naked under any circumstances. First, he should be wearing a diaper to protect both of you from becoming wet. Moisture will have a cooling effect on your skin and his skin. A standard preemie diaper is often too large on a very small baby. If you do use one make sure it is folded down so skin contact can occur from his belly button up. Try a surgical mask instead of the diaper for a really small baby.

Purchase a soft, lined woolen hat rather than using the standard issue stockinet cap given by the hospital. The greatest heat loss in your baby is lost through the head. A new flannel receiving blanket works best to cover your baby. Start with the blanket folded in fourths. Should your baby become too warm, first take off the head cap and booties, and then you can unfold the blanket once and then twice.

Tiny or sick babies may be unable to keep their chests expanded during upright Kangaroo Care. If your preemie is under 32 weeks and weighs less than 1,500 grams or if she is very sick, you will need to hold her in a more reclined position. Angle her so that she's resting on one breast or the other. Also use a blanket that has been previously warmed. If your baby is still on a ventilator, recruit two staff members to assist you in getting your baby into position. Your chair must be close enough to the equipment so that the wires and tubes are not pulled or stretched. Have everything set up with you in the chair before you arrange the transfer. A semi-reclined position is best for both of you, allowing your baby's head to be turned in one direction or the other so that the ventilator tubes and gadgetry rest on your shoulder.

Place your baby, skin-to-skin, on your chest placing your baby in the fetal position, arms and legs bent and tucked beneath the torso to help conserve your baby's heat. Your breast will heat up or cool down your baby automatically as needed. Close access to your breast will give your baby the most practice with breastfeeding. Your baby will eventually suck and rest and suck and rest as needed. Ask for special assistance from your health team as premature infants have common problems with breastfeeding that can be easily remedied with help.

Stay in place for as long as you feel comfortable. Even thirty minutes of Kangaroo Care can have a tremendous positive impact on both you and your baby. Expect your baby to fall into a long deep sleep. You may want to use this time to nap as well. Most sessions last an hour or two. Some mothers are choosing to wear their babies day and night for the first month or so with excellent results for both parents and baby.

Enlist the support of your partner. Men receive the same benefits as we do and are often surprised at their own nurturing abilities and they begin to feel deeply attached to their tiny babies. The best time to begin Kangaroo Care is immediately after birth. Talk to your health team about this great new advance in premature care and let them know of your intention to Kangaroo Care your baby. You may want to work on changing the environment of your hospital's Intensive Care Nursery to further help your baby to sleep and grow:

1.  Ask to have the lights dimmed.
2.  Have the radio turned off and have your baby placed furthest away from traffic.
3.  Ask for a smaller private or semi-private room for your baby.
4.  Have the nurse put up a "Please do not disturb me. This is my nap time" at designated times of the day and night that you choose.
5.  Make a sleep shade (like a sun shade) to help facilitate your baby's day-night cycling. Allow it to cover the top and two sides of the incubator but leave open the ends from which the wires emerge.
6.  Create a nest for your baby within the incubator or crib. You can use bolsters of fabric that are at least as high as his body. There are various ways of creating these bolsters. You can use rolled blankets, foam forms, rubber doughnuts, a hammock, Neocrate by Snugli or even a bean bag that you've made the size of your baby and covered with a soft natural fabric.
7.  Ask the hospital to have a "nursery shutdown" when all babies are given a long opportunity to sleep undisturbed.

Nursery shutdown, reduced lighting, and sleep shades are examples of conditions you can implement or advocate to protect your infant from the stressful NICU environment. Distancing your baby from sudden loud noises and nesting her will reduce her agitation. Day-night cycling, prone positioning and nesting all foster better sleep as does Kangaroo Care. Kangaroo Care also has the potent role of replacing noxious experiences with pleasant loving ones."

Reprinted with kind permission: Kangaroo Care: The Best You Can Do To Help Your Preterm Infant by Susan M. Ludington-Hoe PhD with Susan K. Golant.

# What You Need To Know Before You Have Your Baby: Exposing the Secrets About Circumcision

"There was a well-kept secret I wish I'd known before my babies were born. Sadly, I didn't learn about circumcision until my sons were 10, 17, and 20 years old. Prior to their birth, there was no "informed consent," there was simply, "It doesn't hurt, only takes a minute, and will protect your son from a myriad of ills that will befall him if he isn't circumcised." I was consenting to something that would be good for my sons, something medically sound, or so I thought.

Then, as a nursing student in 1979, I became truly informed. I witnessed a circumcision, an event that literally changed the course of my life. As I watched a newborn baby, arms and legs strapped spread-eagle to a plastic board, struggle against his restraints and heard him frantically scream with the agony of having the most sensitive part of his penis cut off without pain medication, I began to cry. The doctor looked at me and said, "There is no medical reason for doing this!" That remark led me to research a subject I should have investigated 10, 17, and 20 years earlier. I'll share the basics of what I've learned during these past three decades.

No national or international medical association in the world recommends circumcision, and some, recognizing the harm of this cosmetic surgery performed on nonconsenting minors, have begun to recommend against it.

Circumcision is a primal wound that interferes with maternal/infant bonding, disrupts breast-feeding, and undermines the baby's first developmental task of establishing trust. Circumcision is where sex and violence meet for the first time, leaving a premier and life-lasting imprint of pain between the penis and the brain.

The foreskin is a normal, protective, sexual organ that has several functions. It covers and protects the head of the penis (glans) and the urinary meatus, keeping the urinary tract free from contaminants and the glans soft and moist, as it is meant to be. The foreskin provides the tissue necessary for full expansion of the penis, and it houses approximately 20,000 specialized erogenous nerve endings that allow a male to know what his penis is feeling and where he is in relation to the ejaculatory threshold. During early adult years, the most common complaint of circumcised males is premature ejaculation. Later in life, it's loss of sensitivity, penile dysfunction, and impotence. These are the consequences following amputation of a vital part of the sex organ.

Circumcision, like any surgery, has inherent risks, including hemorrhage, infection, surgical mishap, and even death. Today, with the threat of the deadly hospital and community-associated methicillin-resistant Staphylococcus aureus (CA-MRSA), notably higher among circumcised baby boys, it is crucial to protect babies from non-therapeutic open wounds.

Circumcision is painful—even when analgesia is used. The only effective analgesia requires four painful injections into the penis. After circumcision, a baby urinates and defecates into the raw wound for the week to ten days it takes to heal, causing additional pain and trauma.

Circumcision leaves both physical and psychological scars, denies a male's right to a fully functioning penis, leaves him with decreased sensitivity, pleasure, and sexual fulfillment, and it undermines his right to self-determination.

Circumcision is always fear-based. The fears have changed over the years, some persisting long past the time the myths were debunked. While the origins of circumcision as a puberty rite or religious ritual are lost in history, we know very well how and when circumcision was medicalized and the fears that have perpetuated it..

During the mid1800s in the English speaking countries (starting with England), people believed disease was caused by masturbation. These diseases included scoliosis, hernia, gout, kidney disorders, blindness, epilepsy, masturbatory insanity, and more. Cutting off the best part of the external genitals of males (the foreskin) and females (the clitoral hood and the clitoris), was adopted to prevent masturbation and, therefore, disease.

With the development of the microscope and a new theory of disease, the germ theory, the next excuse for circumcision was to rid the penis of germs. Then, the foreskin itself was maligned as dirty, but only where circumcision was practiced.

The dreaded disease of the 1930s was penile cancer; in the 1950s, it was cervical cancer; and, in the 1960s, with the sexual revolution, it was sexually transmitted diseases. Circumcision was purposed to prevent them all.

During the 1970s, as people questioned and challenged certain routine medical procedures—radical mastectomy, tonsillectomy, episiotomy, and circumcision—a new fear-based tactic was introduced: a boy needed to look the same as dad and peers. This excuse was never mentioned when circumcision was instituted and sons of intact fathers were circumcised.

During the 1980s, urinary tract infections became the excuse to circumcise but, if antibiotics are successful in treating UTIs in baby girls, obviously that works for boys, too. And, less than two percent of babies, boys or girls, get UTIs.

During the 1980s, circumcision to prevent HIV/AIDS was proposed, however, the USA has one of the highest AIDS rates and one of the highest male circumcision rates in the developed world, so it obviously doesn't work. There is no need to resort to expensive, risky circumcision when aggressive educational programs about the danger of HIV, the importance of safe sex and condom use, and dispensing free condoms have proven successful. Programs promoting circumcision should be questioned and challenged.

The Declaration of the First International Symposium on Circumcision acknowledges the unrecognized victims of circumcision and, in support of genital ownership rights of infants and children, states: We recognize the inherent right of every human being to an intact body. Without religious or racial prejudice, we affirm this basic human right. Due to the lifelong consequences of the permanent surgical alteration of children's genitals, it becomes imperative that children have the right to own their own reproductive organs and to preserve their natural sexual function."

Marilyn Fayre Milos, RN, is co-founder and Executive Director of NOCIRC and coordinator of the International Symposia on Circumcision, Sexual Mutilations, and Genital Integrity. She has co-edited five books of symposia  proceedings, including Sexual Mutilations: A Human Tragedy, Male and Female Circumcision: Medical Legal and Ethical Considerations in Pediatric Practice, Understanding Circumcision: A Multidisciplinary Approach to a Multidimensional Problem. She is also the editor of the NOCIRC Annual Newsletter. She is the recipient of the California Nurses Association's Maureen Ricke Award (1989) for having "raised public consciousness about America's most unnecessary surgery" and her "dedicated and unwavering commitment to 'righting a wrong.'" She also received NurseWeek magazine's "Nursing Excellence 2001" award "For outstanding advocacy for the past 22 years on behalf of those among us who are the most vulnerable and unable to protect themselves -- infants and children." She is a Diplomate of the American Board of Sexology. NOCIRC, PO Box 2512, San Anselmo, CA 94979-2512 Tel: 415-488-9883 www.nocirc.org.

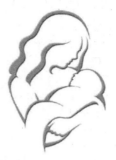

# Chapter Eight - Eighth Month

As your baby becomes heavier, make sure you take every opportunity to sit rather than stand. Do not lift heavy items. Take the elevator instead of the stairs and continue to remind those around you that you are pregnant and that some activities are not advised.

Keep a supply of ice cubes and crushed ice to suck on. You can also freeze lemonade in your ice cube trays.

Anyone who offers to help now in the first few days after your baby's arrival – accept! Even having a load of laundry done or the house tidied up a bit is a wonderful break. Also having someone to talk with will help you to recuperate emotionally as well. Ask what they do best and book them in advance. Remember you should be the one handling your baby, as parenting is practice. Have your helpers take care of the one hundred and one other tasks that need to be done once a new baby is in the house.

Gardening is a great stress reliever and squatting while weeding strengthens your thighs and pelvic floor, to assist you with the pushing phase of your delivery.

Try to relax! Take time out each and every day to do something for yourself. Your body needs time to rest and sometimes a nap is not always possible (especially if you have older children or if you are working throughout your pregnancy). Time for yourself is very important for your health and your state of mind.

## Preventing Postnatal Depression

Purchase extra prenatal vitamins and minerals from your health food store. You will need to continue your prenatal vitamins for at least ninety days after your baby is born to help you get back into pre-pregnancy shape.

Stock your cupboards and freezer with easy to prepare meals and high energy snack foods. Prepare to have enough food put away for your first two weeks of rest. Arrange for a caretaker for yourself for the first two weeks. You will require someone to prepare food, take trips to the drug store and grocery store, and to watch the baby while you take walks outside, bath or sleep.

Drugs used to induce or speed up your labor can cause prolonged postnatal depression. Avoid these drugs during childbirth for this reason alone.

Plan to have telephone contact with someone who knows you throughout your first month home. Depression can silently sneak up on you and those who know you well, will become aware of it often before you even realize that you are depressed.

It is important to grieve for what you have lost: independence, money, time for your own interests, self-care, and freedom to come and go as you please or whatever you feel is missing from your life now. You may also be grieving the end of your pregnancy. Be mindful of what you have gained in exchange.

Some days will be easier than others.

Make sure you are continuing to take your prenatal vitamins. B vitamins are extremely helpful in combating depression.

St. John's Wort, an extract from a flower, is the newest natural product to assist in healing postnatal depression. It can be purchased at any health food store in capsules, drops or oil. Taking 300 milligrams three times a day has given many women quick relief from depression. It is a natural and non-toxic product and can be taken while you continue breastfeeding.

Talk to other women who have just had babies. You will be surprised to find out that they are having many of the same feelings that you are.

If you had a bad experience during your birth find a way to heal this. One of the best ways is to vent your feelings to your health team. Let them know what you feel they could have done differently. You may not be able to change your experience, but you may change the experience of those who come after you. Talk about your feelings with those around you. Be ready to let others step in to help so that you can have time to yourself to rebalance.

Make sure that you are getting out of the house on a regular basis to reconnect with your friends and family. Take up all offers for baby-sitting even if it's just for an hour or two.

It is very important that you seek medical advice for all prenatal and postnatal symptoms of depression. There is no need to be embarrassed or to feel stigmatized if you are not emotionally feeling good about yourself or your baby at any stage of your pregnancy.

This Isn't What I Expected: Recognizing and Recovering from Depression and Anxiety after Childbirth by Karen R. Kleiman, MSc, and Valerie D. Raskin, MD, is a book for the one out of four mothers who find life after a baby unexpectedly difficult for a variety of reasons.

This book provides excellent information on how to recognize the signs, where to find help and everyday coping techniques. Several exercises are designed to help you explore your feelings about parenthood, how you were parented, and how your expectations have clashed with reality. The real-life stories help us to see ourselves through others and know that we are not alone.

If you feel that you can't cope, or if you have feelings of violence towards yourself or your baby, seek professional help immediately. Don't wait to feel better: if you have a clinical depression it will most likely get worse with time so deal with this situation right away. Your closest childbirth association, doctor or midwife will be able to direct you to an agency that has experience with prenatal or postnatal depression.

## Preparing for a Gentle and Easier Labor

You may be able to avoid the pain of back labor during delivery by assisting your baby to turn to the proper placement, head down and facing back, by going on your hand and knees in the evening and gently rocking your hips back and forth. Place your knees apart to open up the pelvic area. You can also lean against an ottoman or the sofa if this is more comfortable. This position will help by giving your baby more room to turn around and this position is soothing for yourself as well. A ten-minute session of this every other night is plenty.

Visualize your baby actually turning in your womb, head down with the face back. Every time you go in for your prenatal appointments look at your doctor's charts and models of babies to clearly see the position your baby will need to be into for an easy birth.

If your heath team says your baby has dropped and you still have a few weeks to go until your due date – celebrate! The longer your baby is "engaged" the more pliable your body becomes.

A little pressure for a longer time will make dilating during active labor quicker and easier. Some babies do not "drop" until the last few moments of delivery, so don't be concerned if you don't feel this happening.

# Preparing for Breastfeeding Your Baby

Most women, around the world, are breastfeeding again. Over 85% of women breastfeed their babies. Breastfeeding is a learned skill, like riding a bike, skating, or driving a standard shift vehicle. This is a good time to begin reading up on breastfeeding, creating a support network, and understanding why your breast milk is so important for you and your baby.

## Breastfeeding Facts

- Breastmilk is free.
- Breastfeeding is natural.
- Breastmilk is the best food available for your baby.
- Breastfeeding will create a strong bond of love and trust between you and your baby.
- Breastfed babies cry less.
- Breastfed babies are calmer.
- Breastfed babies have colds of a much shorter duration, if any.
- Breastmilk can easily be frozen and stored for future use.
- Breastfed babies always receive the right amount of milk.
- Breastfed babies are easily taken with you.
- Breast size has no correlation to the amount of milk you produce.
- Breastfed babies are more secure.
- Breastfed babies have less gas.
- Breastmilk contains natural enzymes to help your baby easily digest each meal.
- Breastfeeding will not change the shape of your breasts, pregnancy can.
- Breastmilk provides all the nutrition your baby requires for the first six months of life. You do not have to supplement breast milk with any other food during this time. You will continue to produce breastmilk for as long as you choose to breastfeed.
- Some mothers are continuing to breastfeed their children into the second year and beyond to boost their children's immune systems. Breastmilk contains hundreds of antibodies that strengthen your baby's immune system.
- Breastmilk triggers the mothering hormone, prolactin, with every feeding causing you to feel more relaxed and attached to your new baby.
- Breastfed babies have better tooth and mouth development.
- Breastfeeding comforts you and your baby emotionally.
- Breastfeeding is convenient and economical.
- Breastfeeding can help you to have a lower incidence of breast cancer.

- Breastfeeding tones the muscles of your uterus and helps your body recover and recondition itself more rapidly.
- Breastmilk is ready when your baby is.
- Breastmilk changes its consistency throughout each feeding and will change to meet the needs of your baby as your baby grows.
- Breastmilk is the best milk for premature infants.
- Breastfeeding provides resistance to ear infections.
- Breastfeeding can help to prevent or forestall allergies and asthma.
- Breastmilk will cool or warm for your baby automatically.
- Breastmilk easily increases to meet the demands of your growing baby.
- Breastmilk is always sterile, clean and ready.
- Breastmilk can reduce celiac, crohns and colitis bowel diseases.
- Breastfeeding can reduce diabetes, pneumonia, obesity, meningitis, cirrhosis and lymphoma in your baby.
- Breastmilk is the best choice for every baby.

## Secrets to Successful Breastfeeding

Is there a secret to successfully breastfeeding your baby? Maybe just one! Be prepared to spend all of your time breastfeeding! At least it may seem like this in the first two weeks. The key to the first month is to breastfeed whenever your baby is hungry, which usually means whenever they are awake. You may be breastfeeding every two hours during the first few days after your milk comes in. After the first few weeks you will have established your milk supply to suit your baby and you exactly and then you can relax. After the first month your baby will also become more proficient and each feeding becomes faster.

Many mothers are continuing their breastfeeding relationship with their babies when they return to their careers. You can breastfeed your baby in the mornings, the evenings and on the weekends. Once your breastfeeding has been established you will continue to produce breast milk. Some babies will change their feeding schedules around to take full advantage of you when you are available and have a heavier feeding demand during the evening rather than the day.

How do you relax when breastfeeding? It is hard to feel comfortable if you think everyone is watching you when you feed your baby. Find a quiet spot (in public or private), cover your baby and yourself with a large soft blanket and tune out your surroundings as best you can. This will take a little practice, but once you have it mastered, you will find being able to nurse anywhere, anytime is a real bonus.

When at a shopping mall you can go into any changing room in a department store, many malls now have special mother's rooms or you can go to your car for some peace and quiet for breastfeeding. Once you've had some practice you may find that you can easily breastfeed anywhere without attracting any attention at all. Just make sure you are pulling up your top rather than undoing the buttons to keep your chest covered. At a party ask to use an empty bedroom if you like. In your home set up a private space with your rocker and footstool and a small table for books, telephone, a glass of juice or water and high energy snacks. Let everyone at home know that this is your spot for breastfeeding and that you will defend your territory.

Wearing nursing-accessible clothing is a must. Two-piece outfits work best; pants and a T-shirt, a skirt and blouse, tights and long sweaters. It is difficult to breastfeed your baby in the wrong clothing. Remember to wear two-piece outfits to bed. It can get cool in the middle of the night so keep a housecoat at the foot of your bed or within easy reach.

People ask a lot of questions when you are breastfeeding. "Does it hurt?" "Aren't you embarrassed?" "Wouldn't a bottle be easier?" Try to answer them honestly and openly. They are just curious. Answer these questions with a smile and tell whoever asks why you've chosen to breastfeed. Satisfy their curiosity. After all, the more people who are educated about breastfeeding, the more support there will be for everyone.

How do you keep siblings entertained while breastfeeding? Breastfeeding is especially time-consuming in the first few weeks, and an older brother or sister may feel left out of the loop. One of the best things you can do while breastfeeding is to read to the older children. Have the older child sit beside and turn the pages when you "beep." This also has a calming effect on your baby, as the older child is not running about pleading for attention.

How do you keep your partner involved if you are doing all the feeding? Let your partner know that you will be expressing milk and freezing it to create a milk bank that any member of the family can access to feed the baby. In the first few weeks after the birth of your baby you will have an abundance of milk, making this an excellent time to start your own milk bank. Have your partner choose his favorite baby task and have him be in charge of that activity. Set up a special time in the evening for them to enjoy their activity or task together.

Sleeping when your baby sleeps is a tried and true method to combat exhaustion. Doing housework during this period will add to the natural tiredness you may be feeling. Save the housework for when your baby is up and alert; you can easily place your newborn in a portable infant seat for company while you go about your tasks. In the first few months you must guard your energy, and having one or two short naps during the day or early evening will recharge your batteries. Ask for help with the laundry, cooking, shopping and whatever else you need.

Older children can spend quiet time in their rooms every day. Keep in mind that this quiet time may sometimes be at odd hours, but it is quiet time, nonetheless. If they are old enough, they can understand that quiet time is not always just after lunch, but may come at 2:30 when the baby's sleeping. Set the kitchen timer to wake you up in 45 minutes so that the older child is not left in their room for too long.

Breastfeeding your baby can make you hungry and thirsty. Make up a tray of mini-muffins, healthy cookies or fruit. Something you can grab (with one hand) in the middle of the night. A shot of milk, juice or water helps to fight dehydration, which you may feel at night. Keep these items within easy reach. Snacking while you breastfeed your baby can also assist in fighting fatigue. Keep bottles of water in the car and one in your purse.

Consider breastfeeding for at least a one-year period or longer to give your baby an excellent immune advantage.

## Breastfeeding Clinics

Plan to attend a breastfeeding class or a La Leche support group now in your neighborhood. It is important that you find out how to breastfeed your baby before birth. There is a lot of information that can make your breastfeeding experience a success for you both from the start. Meet the instructor so you will always have someone to call upon should the need arise. Most of the moms who volunteer with this organization overcame some challenges themselves during breastfeeding and usually have great empathy for any concerns or questions you may have.

## Breastfeeding Is Priceless - There Is No Substitute for Human Milk

The World Health Organization, health care associations, and government health agencies affirm the scientific evidence of the clear superiority of human milk and of the hazards of artificial milk products. The World Health Organization recommends that mothers exclusively breastfeed their infants for at least the first six months, continuing breastfeeding for two years and beyond.

1 Human milk provides optimal benefits for all infants, including premature and sick newborns. The American Academy of Pediatrics encourages pediatricians to promote, protect, and support breastfeeding in their individual practices as well as in hospitals, medical schools, communities, and the nation.

2 Although more US mothers are initially breastfeeding their infants, in 2001 less than half of mothers who initiated breastfeeding did so exclusively (without supplementing with artificial milk or cow's milk) and less than one in five were breastfeeding exclusively at 6 months.

3 A Healthy People 2010 goal is to have three-quarters of mothers initiate breastfeeding at birth, half of them breastfeed until at least the fifth or sixth month, and one-fourth to breastfeed their babies through the end of the first year.

4 Human milk is unique. Superior nutrients and beneficial substances found in human milk cannot be duplicated. Breastfeeding provides optimum health, nutritional, immunological and developmental benefits to children and protection from postpartum complications and future disease for mothers.

# Benefits of Breastfeeding for Children

### Enhanced Immune System and Resistance to Infections.

- The infant's immune system is not fully mature until about 2 years of age. Human milk contains an abundance of infection fighting factors that are transferred to the child, including agents that act against viruses, bacteria, and intestinal parasites.
- Breastfeeding reduces the incidence of respiratory infections, ear infections, pneumonia, diarrhea, and urinary tract infections.
- Breastfeeding helps protect against sudden infant death syndrome (SIDS).
- Human milk contains factors that enhance the immune response to polio, tetanus, diphtheria, and influenza.

## Protection Against Chronic Disease

- Exclusive breastfeeding for a minimum of four months decreases the risk of Type I diabetes (insulin- dependent diabetes mellitus) for children with a family history of diabetes.
- Exclusive breastfeeding for a minimum of four months decreases the incidence of asthma and eczema.
- Anti–inflammatory factors in human milk reduce the incidence of bowel diseases such as Crohn's disease and ulcerative colitis.

- Breastfed children are less likely to develop Hodgkin's disease or leukemia in childhood.

## Nutritional, Physical, and Mental Benefits

- Human milk is the ideally balanced and easily digested form of infant nutrition. Human milk is less stressful on immature infant kidneys and contains lipids and enzymes that promote efficient digestion and enhance nutrient absorption.
- The composition of human milk changes over the course of a feed, the day, and over time to accommodate the changing needs of the growing child.
- Breastfeeding reduces the risk of childhood obesity. Breastfed children gain less weight and are leaner at one year than formula-fed children.
- Human milk contains long-chain polyunsaturated fatty acids important for brain growth.
- School age children who were breastfed score higher on cognitive and IQ tests and tests of visual acuity.
- Breastfeeding decreases the incidence of dental cavities and the need for orthodontistry.

## Benefits of Breastfeeding for Premature Infants

- Mothers of premature infants produce milk that is higher in protein and other nutrients than milk produced by mothers of full-term infants.
- Human milk contains an enzyme that helps the baby digest fat more efficiently.
- Breastfeeding premature infants helps protect them against gastrointestinal and infectious disease.
- Human milk enhances brain stem maturation in premature infants and raises childhood IQ test scores.
- Breastfeeding the premature infant reduces hospital costs and length of hospital stay.

# Benefits of Breastfeeding for the Mother

- Women who start breastfeeding immediately benefit from an increased level of oxytocin, a hormone that stimulates uterine contractions lowering the risk for postpartum bleeding.
- Women who breastfeed are more likely to lose their pregnancy weight and less likely to become obese.
- Breastfeeding reduces the risk of ovarian and pre-menopausal breast cancer, heart disease, and osteoporosis. The more months women

breastfeed over their lifetime, the greater the protection.

- Exclusive breastfeeding delays the return of the menstrual cycle for 20 to 30 weeks and may lower the risk of anemia.

## The Cost of Not Breastfeeding

- US families spend $2 billion a year on human milk substitutes such as artificial milk otherwise known as formula.
- It costs an additional $1.3 billion dollars to cover sick-child office visits and prescriptions for respiratory infections, ear infections, and diarrhea in non-breastfed infants during the first year.
- In the first year of life, it will cost more than $25,000 to treat lower-respiratory infections in 1,000 never- breastfed infants compared with 1,000 infants exclusively breastfed for at least three months.
- The excess cost of treating Type I diabetes (insulin-dependent diabetes mellitus) in formula-fed children is more than $1 trillion.
- Private and government insurers spend a minimum of $3.6 billion a year to treat medical conditions and diseases preventable by breastfeeding. Formula has a long history of recalls for bacterial contamination or mis-manufacture that have in many cases resulted in instances of illness, permanent injury, or death. Information on formula recalls is available at: http://www.salerts.com/rcls/category/child.htm.

Reprinted with the kind permission of The Coalition for Improving Maternity Services(CIMS). For further information about The Coalition for Improving Maternity Services contact www.motherfriendly.org.

## Child Care

Begin to investigate your child care options. All daycare centers have a limit of infants that they can accept, so booking ahead will help with this. Some daycare centers offer subsidies from the government which can reduce the amount you pay. Ask in advance about subsidies and fill out the necessary paperwork so that you have it on hand. Overtime is often charged at double, so make sure you are clear about this at the start. Taking the time now to investigate what is offered in your city will help you to make calm, clear decisions after your baby arrives.

Take a look at the amount you actually bring in from working after taxes, daycare, transportation, lunches, extra clothing expenses and all costs associated with working. Are you actually getting ahead?

Studies are showing that the first three years of your baby's life is the most critical period of time and when you can make the greatest impact in your baby's life. This is the time when your baby will develop the framework and foundation of who he or she will become. Giving up some material benefits now in exchange for this extremely important time in your baby's life may be the most rewarding option you can choose.

Some mothers find it very difficult to spend extended time away from their careers and do not feel a great deal of satisfaction with remaining at home on a full time basis. If this is your personality, then you will need to set up an excellent support system of people to assist in caring for your baby. Perhaps working from home, your partner taking care of baby or working on a part-time basis can be arranged for the first year or two of your baby's life.

Many mothers do not have the option of either working full time or staying home full time. For those mothers, being actively engaged with your baby when you are together can give you good results. Learning new skills like Baby Language and Baby Signs can help you to more easily engage with your baby when you are together.

Whatever your personality style and preferences for raising your child whether by choice or having no choice, look for the situation that is the most positive for both mother and baby for the best results.

## Siblings

Spend time with older children prior to your baby's arrival discussing what it will be like to have a new baby in the house. Many children think they will have a ready-to-play friend arriving. The older children need to understand that babies eat, sleep, cry and take up a lot of Mom and Dad's time and energy in the first few months. Their expectations will be more realistic if they are prepared in advance for these events.

If you are planning a home birth or family-centered birth, explain that labor does hurt, and give them an idea of what the new baby will look like and act like at birth. Most children handle a home birth with tact and diplomacy and can provide great comfort to their mother during labor and birth. Allowing the children to come in and out of the room as they please and having a responsible adult on hand to care for them during the birth can help them to participate in this exciting day. Mothers who birth at home are reporting that there is less friction and sibling rivalry in the family due in great part to the children's involvement in the birth.

# Planning a Waterbirth

In the past decade or so, women from all walks of life have labored and given birth in such unusual water containers as a skip in England and glass tanks in Russia. Women have given birth in hot springs and in the sea, in swimming pools, paddling pools, Jacuzzis, in ordinary baths and purpose-built tubs all over the world.

Waterbirths have captured women's imagination as a natural, safe and effective method of pain relief, as part of the trend towards natural childbirth. It's an idea whose time has come. Midwives have known about the soothing effects of warm water for generations. The first medically-recorded waterbirth took place in France in 1803. The first attendants were at their wits end to know what to do to help a woman deliver after she had been in hard labor for forty-eight hours. One of the midwives suggested a warm bath, hoping that it might ease her pain. Almost as soon as the exhausted woman got into the bath, the baby was born.

Waterbirth seminars are being organized for midwives and doctors and more hospitals are providing facilities for waterbirths. Research has begun to provide evidence and statistics. Women's enthusiasm for waterbirths is helping to make them more widely available and there's growing official recognition that women should be offered the choice of using water in labor and childbirth. For example, in England, the House of Commons Health Committee on Maternity Services has recommended that hospitals provide birthing pool facilities. Since 1993, more than 70 hospitals in Great Britain provide pool facilities to birthing mothers. It's an option that is increasingly available to women in hospitals, homes and birthing centers around the world.

The relaxing effects of water reduce pain during labor and delivery by causing the mother to have a lower heart rate and blood pressure, lower respiratory rate, lower blood lactic acid levels, a decrease in oxygen consumption, lower muscle tone, lower blood cortisone levels, increase in perfusion of internal organs, increase in skin temperature and causes an increase in the electrical resistance of skin.

Warm water also helps the uterine muscle to work more efficiently, it relieves uncomfortable positions, boosts pain relieving endorphins, lowers stress hormones and relaxes pelvic floor muscles helping to stretch the birth canal without tearing and for dilation to occur at a faster rate. Any gentle childbirth will enable you and your baby to feel relaxed and peaceful as you get to know each other, but water does seem to add an extra dimension, a stronger sense of serenity. This may be the effect of the potent emotional, spiritual and symbolic quality of water because in both a literal and symbolic sense, water is the mother of us all. Literally, life on earth first evolved from the sea and, symbolically, water is widely recognized as epitomizing birth and rebirth. Baptism in water represents rebirth, traditional Chinese medicine calls water the mother of life and Freudian psychotherapists interpret water as both birth and the mother.

Dr. Lichy goes on to cover every aspect of water birthing including its fascinating history, safety, choice of tubs and how to book a water birth as well as useful advice on how to make the most of water throughout labor and during delivery. This book is filled with photographs of calm, alert babies and their mothers. The Waterbirth Handbook is a fascinating documentary on the benefits of water birth.

# Natural Remedies for Yeast Infections

Clear your body of excess yeast now if you are having persistent yeast infections. During the course of any treatment for vaginal yeast it is important to cut out sugar and decrease dairy and bread consumption. Purchase any generic bottle of acidophilus capsules (our friendly bacteria), from the cooler in your health food store. Take two capsules orally a day on an empty stomach. Apple cider baths can also help to restore your balance. If you are prone to yeast infections continue to take the acidophilus capsules orally until the end of your pregnancy and for the first few months of breastfeeding. Always store acidophilus in your refrigerator.

Excess yeast in your system can be transferred to your baby through the birth canal. Yeast can cause thrush in a newborn and will cause problems with breastfeeding. Thrush shows up as white patches inside your baby's mouth and your nipples become extremely sensitive and sore, making breastfeeding difficult and painful. Should thrush become a problem during breastfeeding you and your baby will both have to be treated to eliminate it and the drugs available for this treatment are extremely expensive. As always with any challenge you may experience during breast-feeding, call a La Leche Leader or a Lactation Consultant at your nearest hospital. Always consult other women who have breastfed for breastfeeding challenges. You need someone who has personal experience with breastfeeding. The La Leche leaders are always only a phone call away.

If your yeast infection persists see your doctor for alternate treatment. Some vaginal infections may mimic yeast symptoms but may actually be trichomonas, bacterial vaginosis, gonorrhea, chlamydia or even herpes. A quick test by your doctor will show you the cause of the infection.

# Preventing Yeast Infections

"My first day of work as a medical doctor, a woman walked into my office having suffered from vaginal itching for 20 years. She turned out to have a chronic yeast infection, which eventually she was able to overcome. At various times throughout their lives, many women experience one or more vaginal infections. These highly annoying and even painful infections usually clear up rapidly with treatment. However, an estimated 20% of women go on to develop persistent and recurrent yeast infections.

Of course, the female body has its own defenses against invading yeast cells. The vagina itself is a balanced ecosystem. It is an efficient, self-maintaining and dynamic environment with natural defense mechanisms that keep it healthy, moist and clean. The two most important defense mechanisms are the acid base balance and the cervical secretions. This acid condition of the vagina discourages infections by bacteria and other organisms. Friendly bacteria called lactobacillus acidophilus also help to keep the vagina acidic and resistant to infections.

Certain predisposing factors for yeast infections include use of a birth control pill, pregnancy, use of antibiotics, steroid or anti-cancer drugs, diabetes, the overall state of your health and menopause. Predisposing factors that can also cause recurring yeast infections include warm moist conditions, tight or synthetic clothing, deodorants and sprays, perfumed tampons, perfumed toilet paper, bubble baths with chemicals or perfumes, douching, (pregnant women should never douche), improper toilet habits, vaginal abrasions and sex. Yeast probably can be sexually transmitted, but this has not yet been proven. However, in a large percentage of cases, yeast can also be cultured from the penises of men whose partners have recurrent yeast infections. In these cases, the men may need to take oral anti-yeast medications while their partners are being treated. Even for simple yeast infections, condoms should be used until the woman has completed her treatment.

The main symptoms of yeast infections are usually vaginal discharge and itching of the genital area. The discharge is usually white and varies from being a little to a lot; from being thin and mucousy to thick, curdy and cottage cheese-like with anything in between being possible. The amount of itching also varies but can be severe enough to interfere with sleep and normal activities. Some women notice a characteristic odor suggestive of bread dough or the fermenting yeast smell of beer. Other frequent symptoms are swelling, redness and irritation of the outer and inner lips, the labia, painful sex or painful urination due to local irritation of the urethra.

A woman with a full-blown yeast infection is acutely uncomfortable and requires immediate treatment if possible. If you suspect that you have a yeast infection see your doctor as soon as possible in order to get cultures of the vaginal secretions taken. Other vaginal infections can co-exist or produce a similar picture of signs and symptoms.

Persistent and recurrent yeast infections may be part of a larger picture involving widespread overgrowth of yeast organisms in the whole body. This may cause symptoms affecting every system of the body which may include fatigue, depression, digestive difficulties, menstrual problems, sexual difficulties and infertility, arthritis, chronic skin problems, repeated urinary and vaginal infections, asthma, allergic reactions and chemical sensitivities. Candida overgrowth may also be suspected when a person feels very ill and no cause can be found for his or her problems.

Women are particularly susceptible to Candida overgrowth, especially if they have been exposed to tetracycline for treatment of acne or long-term use of the birth control pill. In children, a chronic yeast infection can show up as hyperactivity, learning disabilities, or even in a few cases autism. In adolescents, Candida can cause depression and severe mood swings. A typical story is a top student who suddenly becomes unable to think clearly or learn, and who becomes suicidally depressed. In one teenage girl these symptoms appeared after just a two-month course of tetracycline for acne. Candida has also been implicated in some cases of teenage anorexia.

If you suspect this generalized type of Candida problem, the first step should be to visit your doctor for a complete history and physical examination including appropriate blood tests to rule out other possible causes of your symptoms such as low thyroid function, other glandular abnormalities, anemia, low blood sugar, viral infections or parasitic infections. It is important to remember that each of these conditions can mimic chronic yeast infections or co-exist with them.

The vagina has a wonderful built in defense system. But in today's fast-paced lifestyle, with its over-reliance on drugs, poor diet and environmental stresses, natural defense systems may be overwhelmed. A simple yeast infection now and then is easy to treat but a chronic yeast infection requires a more thoughtful and thorough approach."

Reprinted with kind permission from: Take Charge of Your Body, Dr. Carolyn DeMarco

## What You Need to Know before You Have Your Baby: New Effective Pain Relief for Labor & Delivery

"One of the most emotionally charged issues in childbirth is how to deal safely and effectively with pain during birth. Epidurals have become so commonplace that most hospitals automatically include them in their standard billing protocol for all vaginal deliveries. The epidural at first appeared to be a magic bullet for pain in childbirth. Many women are still told that the medication used in an epidural is completely safe and that it does not reach the baby. The passage of time, combined with new research has begun to reveal a different picture.

There are actually several kinds of epidurals. The type that most people refer to is, in fact, a lumbar epidural – the administration of a regional anesthetic agent, or a combination of an anesthetic agent with a narcotic and/or antihypertensive, which is injected into the lumbar region of the laboring woman's back by a qualified anesthetic care provider. It is performed by inserting a long needle into the epidural space of the spine, through which a soft catheter is threaded. The needle is then removed and the catheter taped in place. Doses of anesthetic can then be periodically or continuously administered through this catheter.

The mother must lie curled on her side without moving during this procedure, which takes from 20 to 30 minutes to complete and take effect. Once it is in effect, she will be numb from her ribs to her toes, and sensations of pain usually will be eliminated. Epidurals can be strong enough to provide complete loss of sensation and all pain during a cesarean, or minimal enough that the mother can still feel when to push in a vaginal birth. A "walking" epidural is a lumbar epidural in which the dosage of narcotics is higher and the regional anesthetic dosage is lower, creating pain relief without total numbness in the lower body.

The Physician's Desk Reference, a well-respected guide to all drugs, their usage, cautions, and side-effects, states the following about the canine derivatives used in epidurals: "Local anesthetics rapidly cross the placenta and when used for epidural blocks, anesthesia can cause varying degrees of maternal, fetal, and neonatal toxicity. Adverse reactions in the mother and baby involve alteration of the central nervous system, peripheral vascular tone and cardiac function. The following possible maternal side effects include hypotension, urinary retention, fecal and urinary incontinence, paralysis of lower extremities, headache, backache, septic meningitis, slowing of labor, increased need for forceps or vacuum delivery, cranial nerve palsies, allergic reactions, respiratory depression, nausea, vomiting and seizures."

Research done in the last five years on the effects of epidural anesthesia on newborns has shown that epidurals result in lowered neurobehavioral scores in the newborn; a decrease in muscle tone and strength, affecting the baby's sucking ability, which can lead to breastfeeding difficulties; respiratory depression in the baby; greater likelihood of fetal malpositioning; and an increase in fetal heart rate variability, thereby increasing the need for forceps, vacuum, and cesarean deliveries and episiotomies. A review of the literature reports that on average over 70% of women receiving an epidural during childbirth experience some side effects.

Very rare but possible risks of epidurals include trauma to nerve fibers if the epidural needle enters a nerve and the injection goes directly into that nerve; a drug overdose resulting in profound hypertension with respiratory and cardiac arrest and possible death; and central nervous system toxicity resulting from an injection directly into the epidural vein. Other medical interventions, such as IVs, continuous electronic fetal monitoring, the use of additional drugs, bladder catheterization, continuous administration of oxygen, and forceps, vacuum extraction, and episiotomies often become necessary as adjunct medical care to an epidural. Epidurals can prolong a labor leading to the possible need to augment labor with more drugs.

The Physician's Desk Reference repeatedly states that "no adequate and well-controlled studies exist for use of these drugs in pregnant women" and that "it is not known whether these drugs can cause fetal harm when administered to a pregnant woman." Many unnecessary epidurals are the result of a well-meaning health care provider telling the birthing mother that, "It's time for an epidural now." Women in labor are vulnerable, and often easily influenced by the attitudes of those around them. Dr. Jeffrey Illeck, an obstetrician at Cedars-Sinai Medical Center in Los Angeles feels that routine epidurals have "become a way of making the nurse's job in large hospitals easier therefore increasing the number of epidurals that occur. Nurses are extremely busy and often have lost their skills to coach a woman in labor." He also states that, "A lot of the problem is the patient's fear and helping them through these fears."

Anything causing fear in the birthing mother will increase her pain. Despite the fact that we have technology at our disposal, our biology provides us with powerful instincts during birth. The first is the need to feel safe and protected. All mammals will instinctively seek out a dark, secluded, quiet, and most of all, safe place in which to give birth. While birthing, mammals give the appearance of sleep and closed eyes to fool would-be predators, and they breathe normally. Some, those who don't perspire, will pant in order to cool down, but humans will most easily achieve a relaxed state through closed eyes and abdominal breathing. This relaxation slows down the birthing mother's brain waves into what is called an alpha state, a state in which it is virtually impossible to release adrenaline, the "fright-flight" hormone. Physical comfort becomes critical, along with the need to have a nest ready for the baby.

Hospital environments often unintentionally disrupt the birthing atmosphere by introducing bright lights, lots of people, noise, and fear-inducing exams and machines. Put it all together and you have fear, and therefore stress, and stress causes pain. The uterine muscles are beautifully designed to deal quite effectively with danger, fear, and stress in labor. The uterus is the only muscle in the body that contains within itself two, opposing muscle groups – one to induce and continue labor and another to stop labor if the birthing mother is in danger or afraid.

Emotional or physical stress will automatically signal danger to a birthing mammal. Her labor will slow down or stop completely so that she can run to safety. In modern times, this goes haywire. We can't run from our fears. Instead, we may release adrenaline, which causes the short, circular muscle fibers in the lower third of the uterus to contract. These muscles are responsible for stopping labor by closing and tightening the cervix. The result is that we literally stew in our own adrenaline. At the same time that the long, straight muscle fibers of the uterus are contracting to efface and dilate the cervix, the short, circular muscle fibers of the lower uterus are also contracting to keep the cervix closed and fight the labor. The result? The very real pain of two powerful muscles pulling in opposite directions each time the birthing mother has a contraction. The constant presence of a loving, supportive, and trained labor coach, effective education about the birthing process, and a health team and environment the birthing mother can trust can make all the difference in the world.

Unnecessary or preventable pain can also be caused during labor by simple things such as prohibiting the laboring mother from walking, changing position, or moving around freely according to her instincts. Freedom of movement literally supports rotation and alignment, the process by which the baby turns and moves down through the pelvic inlet and outlet. Time-honored birthing traditions have always included walking, changing positions, rocking, and even floating in water. Anything that assists the rotation and alignment of the baby during labor will automatically improve the efficiency of contractions, thereby shortening labor and decreasing pain.

Avoiding unnecessary medical interventions during labor will decrease pain because these interventions actually cause pain themselves, leading to routine epidurals. The use of routine interventions interferes with the natural process of birth, which is inherently safe and effective. How is it possible to know whether medical interventions are unnecessary? The answer is surprisingly simple. If both mother and baby are doing fine during labor, they're unnecessary.

Proper and adequate nutrition during pregnancy and eating and drinking to appetite and thirst during labor can also dramatically decrease pain. Inadequate consumption of complex carbohydrates and water during labor can result in dehydration and low blood sugar, both of which cause more painful and less effective contractions.

A safe and effective exercise program during pregnancy should include aerobic conditioning to provide the mother with needed endurance during labor, as well as pregnancy-specific exercises, which include Kegels, pelvic rocking, and squatting to prepare her body physically for labor. When the mother's body is strong and prepared, pain is decreased. She will have the strength and endurance for pushing in second stage labor, perhaps decreasing the length of the pushing stage and thereby decreasing pain.

Pain During Transition – Choose a position that feels right, relax completely and surrender to and trust the birth process. Use counter-pressure if needed and assure the laboring mother that she is almost through.

Back Labor – Use a hands-and-knees position with your labor coach providing counter-pressure on the painful spot. Walking and changing positions can help to rotate the baby out of the posterior position relieving back labor completely.

Crowning – Nature makes the most difficult moments the shortest. Crowning rarely lasts longer than one to three pushes in an unmedicated birth. By choosing her own birthing position and avoiding the traditional hospital pushing positions, the mother can make crowning far less painful. Squatting widens the pelvic outlet by up to 28% in a pregnant woman and utilizes gravity to assist the birth. Your health care professional can also provide perineal massage or support during the delivery.

Once women are educated about epidurals it becomes clear that avoiding one during childbirth may be well worth it to both mother and baby. By taking responsibility for her health and the health of her baby long before labor begins there are a great many things a mother can do to tremendously improve her chances of successfully avoiding an epidural."

Reprinted with kind permission from Mothering Magazine, The Epidural Express: Real Reasons Not to Jump on Board, written by Nancy Griffin, MA, AAHCC. Nancy Griffin is a Bradley Method natural childbirth educator, a pregnancy-recovery exercise specialist, breastfeeding educator and the owner of Mommy Care Mothering Center in West L.A. USA.

## What You Need To Know Before You Have Your Baby: Pushing for First-Time Mothers

"The expulsion of a first baby from a woman's body is a space in time for much mischief and mishap to occur. It is also a space in time where her obstetrical future often gets decided and where she can be well served by a patient and rested midwife. Why do I make the distinction between first time mother pushing and the second or more time mother, multiparous pushing? The multiparous uterus is faster and more efficient at pushing babies out and the multiparous woman can often bypass obstetrical mismanagement simply because she is too quick to get any.

Let's take a typical scenario with an unmedicated first birth at home. The mother has been in the birth process for about twelve hours. The attendants have spelled each other off through the night. Membranes ruptured spontaneously with clear fluid after eight hours in active phase and mother and baby have normal vitals. There is dark red show (about two tablespoons per sensation) and mother says, "I have to push!" This declaration on the part of the mother brings renewed life to the room. The attendants rally and think, finally, we're going to see the baby. The long wait will be done. We'll be relieved to see baby breathe spontaneously. We can start the clean up and be home to our families. Typically, the midwife does a pelvic exam at this point to see if the woman is fully dilated and can get on with the pushing now. It is common to find the woman eight centimeters with this scenario. The mood of the room then turns to disappointment.

My recommendation with this scenario: Don't do that pelvic exam. A European-trained midwife that I know told me she was trained to manage birth without doing pelvic exams. For her first two years of clinic, she had to do everything by external observation of "signs." When a first-time mother says, "I have to push!" begin to observe her for external signs rather than do an internal exam. Reassure her that gentle, easy pushing is fine and she can "Listen to her body." No one ever swelled her own cervix by gently pushing as directed by her own body messages. The way swollen cervices happen is with directed pushing (that is, being instructed by a midwife or physician) that goes beyond the mother's own cues. It has become the paranoia of North American midwifery that someone will push on an undialated cervix. Relax, this is not a big deal, and an uncomfortable pelvic exam at this point can set the birth back several hours. The external signs you will be looking for are as follows:

- When she "pushes" spontaneously, does it begin at the very beginning of the sensation or is it just at the peak? If it is just at the peak, it is an indication that there is still some dilating to do. The woman will usually enter a deep trance state at this time (we call this "going to Mars"). She is accessing her most rudimentary brain stem where the ancient knowledge of giving birth is stored. She must have quiet and dark to get to this essential place in the brain. She usually will close her eyes and should not be told to open them.

- Does she "push" (that is, grunt and bear down) with each sensation or with every other one? If some sensations don't have a pushing urge, there is still some dilating to do. Keep the room dark and quiet as above.

- Are you continuing to see "show"? Red show is a sign that the cervix is still dilating. Once dilation is complete the "show of blood" usually ceases while the head molding takes place. Then you can get another gush of blood from vaginal wall tears at the point that the head distends the perineum.

- Watch her rectum. The rectum will tell you a good deal about where the baby's forehead is located and how the dilation is going. If there is no rectal flaring or distention with the grunting, there is still more dilating to do. A dark red line extends straight up from the rectum between the bum cheeks when full dilation happens. To observe all this, of course, the mother must be in hands and knees or side lying position.

- I use a plastic mirror and flashlight to make these observations. The mother should be touched or spoken to only if it is very helpful and she requests it.

Involuntarily passing stool is another sign of descent and full dilation. Simply put, where there is maternal poop there is usually a little head not far behind.

Why avoid that eight-centimeter dilation check? First, because it is excruciating for the mother. Second, because it disturbs a delicate point in the birth where the body is doing many fine adjustments to prepare to expel the baby and the woman is accessing the very primitive part of her ancient brain. Third, because it eliminates the performance anxiety/disappointment atmosphere that can muddy the birth waters. Birth attendants must extend their patience beyond their known limits in order to be with this delicate time between dilating and pushing.

Often when the primiparous woman says, "I have to push," she is feeling a downward surge in her belly but no rectal pressure at all. The rectal pressure comes much later when she is fully dilated, but in some women there is a downward, pushy, abdominal feeling. I have seen so many hospital scenarios where this abdominal feeling has been treated like a premature pushing urge and the mother instructed to blow, puff, inhale gas and so forth to resist the abdominal pushing. Such instruction is not only ridiculous but also harmful. A feeling of the baby moving down in the abdomen should be encouraged and the woman gently directed to "go with your body."

When I first started coaching births in the hospital I would run and get the nurse when the mother said, "I have to push." I soon learned not to do this because of the exams, the frustration and the eventual scenario of having to witness a perfectly healthy mother and baby operated on to get the baby out with forceps, vacuum or c-section. I have learned to downplay this declaration from first-time moms as much as possible, both at home and in the hospital. Especially if you have had a long first stage, you will have plenty of time in second stage to get people into the room when the scalp is showing at the perineum.

## Feeling stuck

I recommend that midwives change their notion of what is happening in the pushing phase with a first-time mother from "descent of the head" to "shaping of the head." Each expulsive sensation shapes the head of the baby to conform to the contours of the mother's pelvis. This can take time and lots of patience especially if the baby is large. This shaping of the baby's skull must be done with the same gentleness and care as that taken by Michelangelo applying plaster and shaping a statue. This shaping work often takes place over time in the midpelvis and is erroneously interpreted as "lack of descent," "arrest" or "failure to progress" by those who do not appreciate art. I tell mothers at this time, "It's normal to feel like the baby is stuck. The baby's head is elongating and getting shaped a little more with each sensation. It will suddenly feel like it has come down." This is exactly what happens.

Given time to mold, the head of the baby suddenly appears. This progression is not linear and does not happen in stations of descent. All those textbook diagrams of a pelvis with little one-centimeter gradations up and down from the ischial spines could only have been put forth by someone who has never felt a baby's forehead passing over his/her rectum!

Often the mother can sleep deeply between sensations and this is most helpful to recharge her batteries and allow gentle shaping of the babe's head. Plain water with a bendable straw on the bedside table helps keep hydration up. The baby is an active participant and must not be pushed and forced out of the mother's body until he/she is prepared to make the exit.

For anyone who has taken workshops with Dr. Michel Odent, you will have heard him repeat over and over, "The most important thing is to not disturb the birthing woman." We think we know what this means. The more births I attend, the more I realize how much I disturb the birthing woman. Disturbing often comes disguised in the form of "helping." Asking the mother questions, constant verbal coaching, side conversations in the room, clicking cameras—there are so many ways to draw the mother from her ancient brain trance (necessary for a smooth expulsion of the baby) into the present-time world (using the neocortex which interferes with smooth birth). This must be avoided. A recent article on the homebirth of model Cindy Crawford describes how the three birth attendants and Cindy's husband had a discussion about chewing gum while she was giving birth. Cindy describes her experience: "It was absolutely surreal. There I was, in active labor, and they're debating about gum! I wanted to tell them to shut up, but at that point, I couldn't even talk." (Redbook, March 2000). This was in her own home, and she couldn't control the disturbance that was happening in her first birth. Needless to say, she had a long, painful, exhausting second stage.

Human birth is mammal birth. A cat giving birth to her kittens is a good model to look to for what is the optimal human birth environment: a bowl of water, darkness, a pile of old sweaters, quiet, solitude, privacy and protection from predators. When given this environment, 99.7 percent of cats will give birth to kittens just fine. We spend so much money in North America on labor, delivery and recovery (LDR) rooms and now, adding postpartum, LDRP rooms. Yes, it is advancement that women are not moved from room to room in the birth process, but there is so much more that can disturb the process: lighting, changing staff, monitoring, beeping alarms, exams, questions, bracelets, tidying, assessing, chattering, touching, checking, charting, changing positions and so on.

When midwives come back from the big maternity hospital in Jamaica, they bring an interesting observation about birth. The birthing women are ignored until they come to the door of the unit and say, "Nurse, I have to go poopy." They are then brought into the unit and within twenty-five minutes give birth to the baby. Cervical lips are unheard of. Most times, the head is visible when the woman gets onto the birth table. Her entire eight-centimeter-to-head-visible time is done in the company of the other birthing mothers, and she is cautioned not to go near the midwives until the expulsive feeling in her bum is overwhelming. Cesarean section and instrument delivery rates are very low.

## Reversing the energy

Birth is better left alone and pushing should be at the mother's cues. Having said that, I want to address the exceptions to the rule. After hours of full dilation with dwindling sensations, what if the mother is languishing? The sense of anxiety and fatigue in the room builds, and nothing is served by allowing this to go on too long. Such situations often occur at first births, where the mother insists on having her whole family present. This dynamic is one reason why I forbid vaginal birth after cesarean (VBAC) moms to have spectators at their births. Birth is best done in privacy even if the woman desires on a conscious level to have visitors. In this type of situation the midwife can help by changing the direction of the flow. Normally we think of the baby coming "down and out." In this scenario, nothing is moving. It's a bit like having your finger stuck in one of those woven finger traps. The more the mother attempts to bring the baby down the more tired and tight the process becomes. At this point, it can be helpful to get the mother into knee/chest position and tell her to try to take the baby's bum up to her neck for a few pushes. This will sound like strange instruction but, if she has learned to trust you, she will give it a whirl. Reversing the energy and moving it the opposite direction can perform miracles. After five or six sensations in this position with minimal exertion of the mother, the fetal head often appears suddenly at the perineum. For those of you who know Eastern martial arts, you will understand this concept of reversing directions in order to gain momentum. This is midwife Tai Chi!

## Facing Fear

Psychological factors in birth are a never-ending source of fascination to some birth attendants. I try to keep it simple. My job is to facilitate birth not practice psychology. When I start to be afraid at births, the last thing I want to hear is someone else's fears in addition to mine. This is a natural inclination but not helpful for moving energy and getting babies into the world. I have learned to notice when I'm fearful and respond to my fears by saying out loud to the mother, "Linda, what's your biggest fear right now?"

Linda may take some time but eventually she'll say something that I never imagined she's holding as a fear. Usually it is enough for her to simply express it. Sometimes she needs some reassuring input. I find always that when fear is expressed it begins to disappear or at least lose its grip on the birth. Be bold about addressing fear and uncommunicated worry. One first-time Mom responded to my question "What's your biggest fear right now?" with "I'm afraid I won't be able to open up and let my baby out." As soon as the words were out, her baby gave a big push and the head was visible.

## Linguistics and concepts

Midwives have lots of research support encouraging them to be patient with the second stage and wait for physiological expulsion of the baby. Recognizing ways in which we can support the mother to enter that deep trance brain wave state that leads to smooth birth is imperative. I find it very helpful to have new language and concepts for explaining the process to practitioners. Dr. Odent has taught me to wait for the "fetus ejection reflex." This is a reflex like a sneeze. Once it is there you can't stop it, but if you don't have it, you can't force it. While waiting for the "fetus ejection reflex," I imagine the mother dilating to "eleven centimeters." This concept reminds me there may be dilation out of the reach of gloved fingers that we don't know about, but that some women have to do in order to begin the ejection of the baby. I also find it valuable to view birth as an "elimination process" like other elimination processes- coughing, pooping, peeing, crying and sweating. All are valuable (like giving birth is) for maintaining the health of the body. They all require removing the thinking mind and changing one's "state." My friend Leilah is fond of saying, "Birth is a no brainer." After all "elimination processes" are finished, we feel a lot better until the next time. Each individual is competent to handle her bodily elimination functions without a lot of input from others. Birth complications, especially in the first-time mother, are often the result of helpful tampering with something that simply needs time and privacy to unfold as intended."

Reprinted with kind permission from Gloria Lemay and Midwifery Today, Issue 55, Autumn 2000, www.midwiferytoday.com. Lemay is a Traditional Birth Attendant in Vancouver, British Columbia, Canada and a frequent contributor to Midwifery Today and The Birthkit. Gloria Lemay is an honored and well respected member of the birth community with over twenty three years of experience birthing babies. Gloria has received the following awards for achievement; 2002 Women's Voice Award, 1997 YWCA Woman of Distinction Award in Health, and she is an Advisory Board Member for the International Cesarean Awareness Network. To attend courses or workshops by Gloria Lemay contact her at www.glorialemay.com.

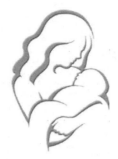

# Chapter 9 Ninth Month – Home Stretch

## Babytime

Around this time you will have increasing prelabor start-stop contractions, you may lose your mucous plug, your water may leak or gush, you may feel your baby's head drop lower in your pelvis giving you more room to breath and you will begin to feel impatient and excited about your baby's impending arrival. None of these signs mean that your labor has actually started. Keep in close contact with your health team during this period letting them know of each new development as it happens.

A first-time mother can labor for days or many hours before going into the delivery stage and moving too quickly to the hospital can frustrate everyone. This is where your professional labor support person can be an invaluable asset to you as she will come to your home when your labor actually begins and can time your departure to the hospital or birthing clinic closely if you will be leaving your home.

This is a good time to:

- Go for a massage.
- Find a family member to walk with.
- Work in your garden.
- Go swimming.
- Take long naps.
- Talk to your baby in the womb. Your baby hears loud noises very well at this stage so explain shower or bath noises, the vacuum cleaner noise, the doorbell or buzzer, telephone ringing and other sounds.
- Babies in utero usually sleep during the day as you rock them to sleep with your movements. If kicking is really getting to you, going for a walk

can rock your baby back to sleep giving both of you a break.
- Eat and drink well to prepare your body and your baby for the upcoming delivery.

Relax and remember that babies are not machines; a normal delivery is between 38 and 42 weeks and longer. Remind your doctor of this should he mention inductions. The more natural your birth, the easier labor and delivery will be for both you and baby. As soon as your doctor or health team intervenes it can set up a chain of events from which there is no turning back. As long as you feel your baby and you are in good health, delay any interventions until you go into natural labor. Watching and waiting at this time can make your labor faster and easier for both you and your baby.

If you are feeling pressure from your team to have your baby by a certain date, get a second and third opinion. Don't buy into the myth that after 40 weeks your placenta won't sufficiently nurture your baby, as long as you continue to eat and drink your placenta will function extremely well. Relax, eat and put your feet up. This is the best time for shopping, finishing the baby's room, and getting organized for your baby's arrival.

Review your birth plan. Have a copy of it in your medical file and discuss it thoroughly with your health care specialists. If you do not reach agreement on your plan, or if you feel uncertain that it will be complied with, it's not too late to change to another caregiver. Make sure you feel confident about your caregiver, follow your instincts completely in this matter, do not let any health professional intimidate you.

If you have time at home get a few things organized for your baby. It goes without saying that your baby's room needs to be prepared and purchases made in that department by now like the crib, clothing items, car seat, receiving blankets and quilts. However, some people forget the obvious, simple things, like diapers and wipes.

Cook ahead! If you have a freezer it is a good idea to get some meals or baking done up ahead of time. Think of yourself being snowed in for a month and plan accordingly. There will be some days during recovery when getting supper to the table will be nearly impossible.

If you are making an announcement in the newspaper, write it up in draft form using the ones in the paper as examples. Then you can just fill in the blanks! Call your newspaper to get rates, deadlines, etc.

If you plan to send announcement cards, buy them ahead of time and address the envelopes. You can fill in the cards once you have the details.

Thank you cards can also be purchased ahead of time so that you can send them to people as the gifts come in. It is rather daunting to have to write 20 or 30 cards all at once. You may find that after your baby arrives you will be too distracted and tired to start from scratch on projects like these.

Go to your health food store and purchase more red raspberry leaf tea. Red raspberry leaf tea will help to condition your uterus for the work it will need to do in the next few weeks. You can use any left-over tea after your baby is born to help shrink your uterus back to its original size.

You'll find a nightly warm bath in clear water a lifesaver for this time of your pregnancy. A bath relaxes tense and strained muscles, soothes away aches and pains and has a very calming effect on both you and your baby. You will also enjoy the feelings of weightlessness.

Short walks by yourself can provide you with the comfort of fresh air, exercise and a great chance to "work out" negative thoughts and become more comfortable with your pregnant body and the baby soon to come.

Find a beauty salon or school offering a package deal for facial, manicure and pedicure. Reward yourself – you deserve it.

## Packing Your Bag

Labor is hard work. Keep your body well nourished on this day. Clothes you will need include heavy socks or slippers for walking, a housecoat, a sweat suit with extra pants to wear home, and perhaps an oversized T-shirt for laboring in. Buy a T-shirt with a funny saying on it to remind you to keep your sense of humor. This is infinitely better than any hospital gown ever designed and will make sure that you can keep some sense of privacy if you require it.

Bring high-energy foods such as a nut mix, chocolate, yogurt, soup and sandwiches and plenty to drink like herbal teas, juice, and non-caffeinated pop. Your camera with flash, birth plan, jumper for baby, hat, baby blanket and an infant car seat will be needed.

A surprise bag with your favorite music, a favorite photograph, and a favorite pillow and blanket can make your room more comfortable and will also help you with the various stages of your labor.

Pack some pain control techniques you have written on separate pieces of paper and placed into an envelope. Have your partner put some jokes or funny sayings in the envelope. Throughout your labor take one out and do what you've written every so often, for example:

Use Picture to Focus On / Play Music / Shower / Walk / Massage / Jokes

/ Loose Lips = Loose Cervix (Dilation occurs faster when mouth is relaxed) = Time for a Kiss / Anything else you can think of.

# Shopping Tips

If your baby will have older siblings you may want to prepare them by letting them buy a small gift for the baby – a blanket or rattle for example. In turn, your baby can buy a small item for them such as a book, healthy goodies or crayons. Your new baby will probably be receiving a lot of attention and gifts so it helps to even things out and help the siblings feel included. It also helps to have the older brother or sister help open the baby gifts as they come in.

Purchase a hot/cold gel pack as well as aspirin or Tylenol for fever when your breastmilk comes in. Going to the drug store at 3:00 in the morning for this essential equipment is disheartening with a full fever. Pick up some heavy flow sanitary napkins. You may go through two or three packages after your baby is born.

## What You Need to Know Before You Have Your Baby: The Tree and the Fruit

### An Analogy

"According to traditional wisdom in rural France, a baby in the womb should be compared to fruit on the tree. Not all the fruit on the same tree is ripe at the same time. A fruit that has been picked before it is ripe will never be fit to eat and will quickly go bad. It is the same with a baby. In other words, we must accept that some babies need a much longer time than others before they are ready to be born. If you have some apple trees in your garden, you will listen to your common sense and choose an individualized and selective approach: you will not pick all the apples on the same day.

### The Routine Strategy

What about human babies? Today, all over the world, a routine approach to postmaturity is typically adopted. This aspect of the industrialization of childbirth is rarely, if ever, the subject of discussion. Modern pregnant women are given a very precise due date. Pregnancies are punctuated by routine medical visits, according to an established program. In the age of medicalized prenatal care, the duration of pregnancy is calculated in weeks rather than months, using the beginning of the last period as the main criterion. Long in advance, women are warned that if their babies are not born on a certain date, their labors will be induced. The first result of such attitudes is that in many hospitals more than one-quarter of labors are artificially induced. The other result is that more and more women doubt that they will go into labor without the help of doctors.

An induced labor is more difficult than a labor that has started spontaneously. It usually leads to the need for epidural anesthesia and an oxytocin drip, which more often than not precedes a cascade of interventions, culminating in a vacuum, forceps delivery or an emergency cesarean. The "labor induction epidemic" helps to explain the rising cesarean rates all over the world.

At the root of this epidemic are statistics. When looking at a very large number of births, it is clear that outcomes are optimal when the baby is born between 38 and 40 weeks. The statistics are not as good when focusing on babies born at 41 weeks or after. Such data lead to simplistic conclusions: "If we routinely induce labor whenever the pregnancy has lasted more than a certain number of weeks (41 in many hospitals), we'll eliminate the risks of fetal distress and even deaths related to postmaturity." The risk of death related to postmaturity is not a legend, but it is usually overestimated. It should be balanced with all the risks associated with induction. Is it wise to induce one-quarter of labors, in order to save one baby in thousands? Are more individualized and selective strategies possible? The answer is, "yes."

## Individualized and Selective Strategies

I know from personal experience in a French state hospital that such an approach is realistic. The first step is always to try to determine when the baby was conceived, by listening to what the pregnant woman has to say about her private life, the regularity of her menstrual cycles, and so on. There are countless anecdotes about women adamant that their babies could not have been conceived before a certain date and that the official calculations are incorrect. We must accept that a pregnancy is supposed to be nine solar months from the day of conception.

After that, the principle is simple. If the baby has been in the womb for more than nine months, its condition is assessed on a day-to-day basis. As long as the baby is in good shape, it is possible to wait. From the time daily assessments have started, only the well-being of the baby is taken into consideration, whatever the duration of pregnancy. The most common scenario, by far, is that one day labor will start spontaneously and a healthy baby will be born. If the baby's skin is peeling, it means that it was already postmature.

Several methods may be combined to ascertain that the fetus is not in danger. Firstly, it is easy for a pregnant woman to evaluate daily the frequency of the baby's movements in the womb. When there is a dramatic change, this should be considered a warning. It is also easy for medical staff to perform repeated clinical examinations. However, the so-called non-stress test (electronic fetal monitoring) is useless.(3,4,5) If the size of the uterus is evaluated every day by the same experienced practitioner (using a tape measure), it is possible to detect a sudden reduction in the amount of amniotic fluid. Another option is a daily "amnioscopy"—a simple, cheap and safe way to check that the liquid is clear. A tube the size of a finger is introduced into the cervix and, thanks to an incorporated light, the color of the liquid can be evaluated. As long as the liquid is clear and contains some flecks of vernix, the baby is guaranteed to be in good shape. This test, which I have used extensively for many years, has never been popular in English-speaking countries and tends to be forgotten in continental Europe as well.

Today ultrasound scans may be repeated on a daily basis. As long as there is sufficient liquid in the uterus, the baby is almost guaranteed to be out of danger. These days, most women are offered a great number of ultrasound scans throughout their pregnancy; most of them are useless, compared with what an experienced practitioner can expect from a clinical examination after listening to the mother-to-be. It seems, on the other hand, that many doctors are paradoxically reluctant to repeat scans when the baby might be overdue. This is precisely the time when scans provide precious data that have huge practical implications. Individualized selective strategies might also lead to reestablishing the use of biochemical tests after the so-called due date; a sudden drop in the urinary estriol levels (and other hormones, such as human placental lactogen) is a sign of placental insufficiency. Routine strategies have largely displaced these non-invasive tests.

And what if, suddenly, the baby seems to be in danger before labor starts? In my view, in this case, it is wiser to perform a c-section right away. The priority is to avoid a risky, last-minute emergency intervention. With such a strategy, labor induction will become exceptionally rare and the number of c-sections related to postmaturity will be much lower than if all labors are induced at 41 weeks.

## In Peace

One drawback of the current prevailing strategy is that many women don't spend the last days of their pregnancy in peace. If they have not gone into labor spontaneously, they become obsessed with the date they were given for induction. Their emotional state probably tends to delay the onset of labor. Some try non-medical methods of induction. These women may not realize that any effective method (from acupuncture to nipple stimulation and sexual intercourse) may initiate labor before the baby has signaled its maturity. There is no natural way of inducing labor. Some methods are undoubtedly unpleasant and even dangerous."

Reprinted with kind permission of Dr. Michel Odent © 2004 Midwifery Today, Inc. All rights reserved. This article first appeared in Midwifery Today Issue 72, Winter 2004, www.midwiferytoday.com. Dr. Michel Odent is familiarly known as the obstetrician who introduced birthing pools and home-like birthing rooms. With six midwives, he was in charge of about one thousand births a year at Pithiviers Hospital in France in the 1960s and 1970s and achieved excellent statistics, with low rates of intervention. After his hospital career he practiced homebirths. Odent is a contributing editor to Midwifery Today and author of The Scientification of Love, The

Farmer and the Obstetrician and The Caesarean. Born in France in 1930, Michel Odent studied medicine at the University of Paris, qualifying in general surgery, obstetrics, and gynecology. His innovative leadership of the Obstetrical Unit of a state hospital in the small town of Pithiviers in Northern France from 1962-1986 brought the world to his door. From 1986-1990 he was commissioned by the World Health Organization to report on planned home birth in industrialized countries. After moving to London in 1990, Dr. Odent organized The Primal Health Research Centre and became an itinerant scholar-teacher to groups around the world. He has published more than 50 professional papers and ten books published in 19 languages. He is editor of Primal Health Research, a newsletter on the long-term health consequences of environmental conditions in utero, at birth, and the first year of life. For further information contact www.birthworks.org.

## What You Need to Know before You Have Your Baby: Overcoming Common Labor Challenges

"All that is needed for the majority of labors to go well is a healthy, pregnant woman who has loving support in labor, self-confidence, and attendants with infinite patience. Sadly most women don't have these things, and then even a straightforward labor can become difficult, with rescue maneuvers taking the place of the nurturing that is the basis of good midwifery care.

Women who have their babies in a hospital are more likely to have difficult labors just because they are in a hospital. This is not to say that problems never develop in planned out-of-hospital births, only that they are usually of a kind that can be solved by simple, noninvasive measures. Here are some of the things that can be done to help when difficulties are encountered, so that you, your midwife or doctor, and birth partner can discuss together what action to take.

### You Are Overdue

Most babies are not born on the date they are expected. Generally speaking, it is safer for them to be born after the expected date of delivery than preterm. Although with prolonged pregnancy every hour may seem like a week, and each week a month, a baby will usually be born within ten days of the expected date. If you go past ten days, it may be because you had a long menstrual cycle, ovulated later than you thought, and so conceived later, or because the date based on ultrasound that you were given was incorrect. Gestational age based on the known first day of the last menstruation is more accurate than ultrasound. There is a random error of two weeks with ultrasound.

If you go past your due date, it may be reassuring to make a note of fetal movements. A baby who is moving vigorously is fine, although a baby makes fewer whole body movements in the last few weeks of pregnancy, because there is a tighter fit in the uterus. A healthy baby continues to kick, often when you are resting or lying in the bath. A simple way of keeping a movement chart is to select a time of day when your baby is always at its most active and monitor what is happening during that time.

If you find your baby has quieted down, the most likely possibility is that labor is about to start and, in this case, there may be other signs, such as a rush of energy as you feel the nesting instinct and want to clean out cupboards or finish a work project; the need to empty your bladder frequently; a slight looseness of the bowels – like a minor digestive upset; low backache; a feeling that your baby's head is hanging between your legs like a coconut; and more frequent contractions of your uterus. When movements are much reduced and labor does not start, contact your health team.

If all is well, there is no advantage to inducing labor simply because your pregnancy is prolonged. In fact there are disadvantages in inductions, since it greatly increases the chances of a cesarean section. Enjoy these last unanticipated days of pregnancy with special activities which otherwise you might not have the time for, that restaurant you meant to try, the concert you thought you wouldn't be able to go to because the baby would just be born, a day with a friend, a picnic, a trip to an art gallery or museum, a play or film that you can fit in now, or a browse around antique or craft shops. Don't just sit and wait for the first twinges and brood over what seems by now to be an elephant pregnancy. Soon there will be a baby in your arms.

## You Think Labor Has Started But It Hasn't

Many women have painful contractions that might be the start of labor in the last few weeks before they actually go into labor. This is prodromal labor, and means that changes are taking place in preparation for labor before dialation starts. It is a sign that contractions are beginning to soften and thin out the cervix and push down the baby's presenting part – the part of the baby nearest your cervix, usually the head. Although tiring, this may reduce the length of time you are in labor.

If this happens to you, it is important to get sleep, perhaps with a special bedtime ritual-soaking in a bath with lavender oil, and then having a hot milk drink with honey, and listening to soothing music as you settle down with a hot water bottle in the small of your back or against your lower abdomen.

## Your Water Breaks Before Labor Starts

Ten percent of women have premature rupture of the membranes at term and eight out of ten of these start labor spontaneously within 12 hours, although sometimes a woman has to wait as long as 24 hours before it begins. Premature rupture is more likely when there have been vaginal examinations in the weeks preceding, so that is a good reason for declining such examinations in the last weeks of pregnancy.

When your water breaks, there may be a gush of fluid or a slow trickle. If there is only a dribble of fluid, it is probably the hind waters, the part of the bubble behind the baby's head, that are leaking, and they often reseal themselves after a while. You can ignore it. If there is a gush of fluid, note whether it is clear or stained brown or green. If it is clear, and your baby is already engaged in your pelvis, you do not need to take special action. If it is stained, the baby has emptied its bowels of meconium, a sign that it could be under stress.

You should call your midwife or doctor so that the baby's position can be checked. Often any meconium present is not fresh, which is a sign that the baby was stressed some time ago. If your baby is in a breech position, meconium is squeezed out mechanically as the bottom is pressed down and this is not an indication that the baby is stressed.

An important thing to know when membranes rupture is the position in which your baby is lying. If the baby is head down and the head is low in the pelvis, there is no possibility of the type of emergency occurring when a loop of cord slips down beneath the head. There is a remote chance of this happening if the head is still high, however, or if the baby is lying in a less usual position as in breech or across the uterus. Once your membranes have ruptured, do not put anything inside your vagina or you may introduce infection. There should be no vaginal examinations out of curiosity either. The more vaginal examinations that take place, the greater the risk of infection.

If you wait anxiously for the first contraction, you will be tired out by the time your energy is really needed. So put on a sanitary pad, change it regularly, and go to bed and sleep, do some work around the house or garden, play cards, chess, or Scrabble, listen to music, or watch television. To check that there is no infection, take your temperature every three hours. If there is an infection, you will become slightly feverish, and you should let your caregiver know this. When you empty your bowels, be careful to wipe from front to back, away from your vagina, so that you do not introduce bacteria from your rectum. Don't starve yourself during this wait. You may not want to eat once labor starts, so avoid a long fast now. Have plenty of fluids – fruit juice, tea, or whatever you wish to help replace your fluids, and keep your energy up with snacks of high carbohydrate food, such as pastas, baked potato, and pancakes with syrup. Some midwives suggest taking supplementary vitamin C to build resistance to infection, 250 mg every few hours.

## Prolapsed Cord

A prolapsed cord is an obstetric emergency. It occurs rarely – in 0.3 percent of pregnancies. It happens occasionally in late pregnancy, when membranes rupture prematurely, whether or not a woman intends to have her baby in the hospital. Your midwife will diagnose that the baby's cord is trapped if it can be felt pulsating in your vagina. But sometimes it is too high to feel, and the clue is a marked deceleration in the fetal heart rate, immediately after membrane rupture, when the presenting part is high. Go to the hospital immediately if this happens.

Emergency treatment of cord prolapse is to get into a knee-chest position with your bottom high in the air. Your midwife inserts two clean fingers in your cervix to press the baby's presenting part up and away from the cord. A prolapsed cord is very unlikely to occur during a home birth or in any birthplace where invasive procedures are not practiced. It is usually a consequence of intervention; in particular of rupturing the membranes artificially when the presenting part is very high.

## A Long, Slow Labor

It is difficult to time the onset of labor precisely and although some women are suddenly aware that this is IT, far more experience a gentle lead-in to labor. The arbitrary decision made by some obstetricians that labor must not last longer than 12 hours, or that dilation must proceed by 1 cm per hour, puts the woman under stress and makes her attendants anxious so that they sometimes act unwisely in an attempt to hurry labor along. They may rupture the membranes in order to hasten a slow labor. But if this is done before 4 cm dilation of the cervix it can actually slow down an already slow labor. In a hospital a long, slow labor is often termed failure to progress, (FTP), only because caregivers find the waiting intolerable. Most long labors are simply variations on a theme, and there is an art in adapting to them and not being hassled or discouraged.

If your labor is slow intersperse activity and rest and change your activities frequently. Avoid boredom. Bake a cake for the celebration afterward, soak in a bath, go for a walk, sew or knit – anything rather than lying in bed wondering if there is something wrong because labor is not going faster.

Eat easily digested, smooth foods such as potato puree, soup, mashed banana, ice cream, sorbet, honey sandwiches, or yogurt, and drink plenty of fluids. Raspberry leaf tea has a mild oxytocic action and may help as well.

Move around and keep changing position in order to stimulate uterine activity, and to encourage the baby to descend and rotate with the crown of the head against your cervix. Rock your pelvis, go up and down stairs, and lunge against the wall.

Soak in a bath or have a shower to refresh you and help you to relax.

Empty your bladder every hour and a half to two hours.

A woman in slow labor welcomes quiet, calm reassurance from the attendants. You should not feel under any pressure of time. It is often good to be left alone with your partner.

Explore what happens when you do nipple stimulation or gentle clitoral massage. You can simply get into bed, send everyone away, turn off the light and have a cuddle with your partner for an hour or two.

## Start – Stop Labor

Some labors are slow in a different way. They start and then seem to stop. The uterus contracts weakly or ceases to contract for an interval, then starts again, but may have another phase of inactivity. There may be plateaus like this when nothing much seems to be happening. A start-stop labor occurs most commonly when a woman is admitted to a hospital and her previous regular, strong contractions become spasmodic. The cause is anxiety. The uterus is very responsive to anxiety and this is as true for other mammals as for women. Interference can make any animal's labor more difficult. Bring what is bothering you out into the open and have your birth partner or midwife help you deal with it.

There is a physical cause for some start-stop labors. The baby's head can be in an awkward position and become stuck. Your midwife will monitor the fetal heart regularly and assess the situation. When a baby is awkwardly positioned, moving about and rocking and rolling your pelvis may coax the baby into a better position so that labor can progress. And even when the head is a tight fit, and the baby's descent through the pelvis is delayed, the spontaneous movements a woman makes can assist the uterus to ease the baby's head through the cervix and down the birth canal.

## A Lull at the End of the First Stage

When the baby's head is high and still above the level of the ischial spines there is often a pause at the very end of the first stage of labor. The uterus rests, and everyone else can rest as well. In hospital, during this pause, the decision is often made to set up a Pitocin drip in order to stimulate the uterus into action. Both in hospital and at home it is wiser to wait for descent and rotation of the head to occur, and at the same time give your body a chance to prepare for the active second stage.

Squatting is a good position for initiating contractions and encouraging rotation of the baby's head so that it can press against your pelvic floor muscles. When the head touches nerves in these muscles, the pushing reflex is stimulated, and oxytocin spurts into your bloodstream, causing strong contractions. If you start pushing simply because you are fully dilated and have been told to do so, but do not feel the spontaneous reflex, you can become exhausted with straining, and are likely to push the baby's head down unrotated, with resulting deep transverse arrest, when the baby cannot turn its head to the easiest position for delivery. In most labors this is completely avoidable if a woman is not urged to push too soon and if everyone waits patiently.

## Morale Drops

Most women feel that they can't go on and would like to postpone having the baby when they reach the end of the first stage of labor. These feelings are a sign of progress; for this is transition, the bridge between the first and second stage. If there comes a time in labor when you are discouraged, you need change:
- Change your position or the kind of movements you are making.
- Find a change of scene. Move to another room or go outside.

- Try changing the rhythm of your breathing.
- Ask for a change in the kind of touch you are receiving.
- Have someone new come in and stay with you.
- If you have been in semi-darkness, now light a lot of candles or turn the lights up. If the room is bright, draw the curtains or dim the lights.
- If you have music in the background, change the tape.
- If you have had your eyes closed during contractions, open them now.
- Perhaps you have been silent during contractions. Now open up and make low sounds that go right down into your pelvis.
- Take an opportunity to freshen up. Splash your face with cold water. Have a bath or shower.
- Suck on cracked ice.
- Pep up your energy with a glucose drink or spoonfuls of honey.

## Worries about the Fetal Heart Rate

The important thing about the baby's heart rate is that, if it slows a lot as contractions reach their peak, it should pick up again about 15 seconds after the end of a contraction. If it does this, the baby is receiving plenty of oxygen. Continue to change your position and change your breathing while monitoring the heart beat as this can often remedy matters.

## You Are Hyperventilating

Hyperventilation is the result of breathing in and out fast and furiously. It often happens at the end of the first stage, when contractions are coming at two minute intervals. The woman breathes too heavily and allows no time for the slight pauses that come naturally between inspiration and expiration. You can avoid hyperventilating by keeping your shoulders and throat relaxed, by focusing on the idea of relaxing a little more with each breath out, and by letting your breathing flow rhythmically. Your helpers can breathe with you so that you do not feel so alone.

## You Become Very Tired

Labor is an intense, energy consuming activity, and may be the most strenuous work you have ever done. A woman often feels as if she is on a treadmill of contractions. Have a drink that will adjust your body's electrolyte balance. "Labor Aid" can be made by mixing together 1 quart water, 1/3 cup honey. 1/3 cup lemon juice, 1/2 teaspoon salt, 1/4 teaspoon baking powder and two crushed calcium tablets. Eat something that does not need much chewing and can just slip down. Do not fight the pain. Go right into it instead. Whatever happens during contractions make sure that you are resting completely in each interval between. Remember that you are having a baby. Extra encouragement at this time may give you a fresh heart.

## You Have a Pushing Urge before Being Fully Dialated

A woman may have the desire to push before her cervix is fully open. Pushing hard against an incompletely dilated cervix can make it puffy and swollen so that it actually closes a little. If you want to push and are not yet 10 cm dilated, you may find the following suggestions helpful: Continue breathing. Do not hold your breath, when the longing to push comes, give two quick breaths out followed by one slow breath out, so that there is a steady rhythm of pant, pant, blow, breath in. It sometimes helps if your birth partner holds up a finger in front of your mouth so that you can direct each blow onto it. As soon as the urge leaves you, breathe fully and easily again. If you are in an upright position, this is the time to change it and lie down on your side or be on all fours. If you have to push, do so with an open mouth and breathing out. Let your uterus do the work while you open up.

## You Get No Pushing Urge

A women can have a baby without deliberately pushing it out. Her uterus sees to that. Until there is an irresistible urge to push, it is sensible to avoid pushing by continuing to breathe. There is no need to hold your breath at all. In this way, all the tissues have a chance to fan out smoothly before the ball of the baby's head eases through, with no damage to ligaments, muscles, or skin. Go with your body. When you are free to follow your uterus, the pushing rhythm which it dictates may vary with different contractions. Some pushes are short and others long. Sometimes there is only one push with a contraction, at other times four or five. Even if you feel unsure about what to do, your body knows how to give birth.

## Meconium Is Passed

The bowels of a mature fetus contain meconium, and if the baby is under stress this meconium is expelled in the amniotic fluid. The presence of meconium is a sign of maturity, but it can also mean that the baby is stressed. If the baby inhales meconium, there is a chance that respiratory tract infection can develop. If you are nowhere near birth when meconium is passed, your attendants will probably suggest that you transfer to the hospital so that a pediatrician can be ready to resuscitate if necessary.

If the baby is about to be born and fresh meconium is passed, your midwife or doctor will simply have a mucus extractor ready to suck out meconium gently – even before the baby's body is born, and before the chest has expanded to take the first breath. It will be easier to do this if you stand with your knees bent or are on all fours. Breathe the baby out gently, rather than pushing, and there will be time for your caregiver to suction out every bit of meconium.

## The Baby Is Coming Very Fast

When the second stage is rapid and it looks as if the baby will pop out like a champagne cork, there are several things you can do to slow down the pace and make birth gentler: Adopt an all fours position, or lie on your side, so that your midwife or doctor can guard your perineum with a hand. Do not squat or stand. Breathe the baby out. Guide your baby down with your breathing. Avoid pushing. If you have to push, breathe again as soon as possible. Release your pelvic floor muscles and relax your perineum by opening your mouth and dropping your jaw. If you want to make noises, bellow, groan, or give deep sighs – resonant sounds that go right down into your pelvis. Do not scream or yelp as that will make you tighten up. Listen closely and be guided by your midwife or doctor.

## The Baby Is a Surprise Breech

Occasionally labor is going well and the birth attendants see something emerging that looks like a bald head, and realize, perhaps after meconium is squeezed out, that it is the baby's bottom. This is an undiagnosed breech. Breech labor is like any other labor up to the point when the baby's body slips out. What may then happen is that the head gets stuck. A breech baby should always be delivered gently to avoid injury to the spinal cord, arms and neck. Left to itself, the baby's body uncurls, the uterus keeps the head flexed, and one or both legs drop out, followed by the body and then the head. In a series of 89 breech births delivered by midwives in New Jersey there was not a single case of extended arms and all the babies were fine. Never forcibly pull the legs in a breech birth as this will cause the baby to become stuck when the arms extend.

If you have a surprise breech, adopt a supported, upright position, legs wide apart and knees bent, in order to give the baby's head the most space and to enable gravity to help it slip through. The worst possible position for a breech delivery is lying on your back with legs raised in stirrups. In that position your sacrum and coccyx are pressed up and the dimensions of your pelvic cavity and outlet are reduced. If you squat, you gain an extra centimeter across your pelvic cavity and two centimeters from front to back.

Once you have adopted a half-standing, half-squatting position, leaning on your birth partner in front of you, your midwife or doctor should be positioned behind you, and should simply wait and watch until the baby's body is completely born. The only intervention that may be necessary is to press gently behind the baby's knees if the feet are up over the shoulders. This will stimulate the baby to bend the knees so that they come down. When the legs are extended, they splint the spine, so that it is more difficult for the baby to take the curve of the birth canal.

As you bend your knees and go into a deep squat, holding on to your birth partner, the baby's body will slip out. The cord may slide down too and if it is wrapped tightly around the baby, your midwife or doctor will carefully unloop it, but only very gently, or it may go into spasm. You may feel a confusing, intermittent pushing urge. Avoid pushing if you can until the head is ready to emerge. Let the baby be born by uterine activity alone. This will enable everything to open up and your tissues to spread wide. As soon as the whole body is born, drop forward, legs still wide apart and knees bent, leaning over some furniture or your birth partner so that your back is almost horizontal. This tilts your pelvis so that the baby's nose and mouth are visible, and whoever is catching the baby can aspirate the nose and mouth with a mucus extractor before the head is fully born. A breech baby often begins to breathe once its chest is born, and may inhale mucus from your birth canal. The mucus can block the nasal passages and although most babies are clever at sneezing out anything that is irritating, in this case manual aspiration is a wise precaution.

## Shoulder Dystocia

When a baby is head down, sometimes a big head is born, and then there is a delay in the delivery of the shoulders. Very rarely the shoulders really are stuck; this is known as shoulder dystocia. If your baby's head is born and then nothing happens, move! Movement itself often releases the shoulders. You may choose a hands and knees position and when the next contraction comes, push hard as your helper applies gentle downward traction to the head. The baby sometimes falls out. Another very good position is to stand with your knees as wide apart as possible. If your baby still does not budge, your helper will reach in with two fingers and find the baby's posterior armpit, the one nearest, and either pull the shoulder forward or pull down the arm. A fourteen pound baby can be delivered this way with no need at all for an episiotomy.

## Twins

If you have undiagnosed twins or labor with diagnosed twins proceeds too quickly to risk getting to a hospital: Warm the room and fill hot-water bottles so that the babies will not become cold. Small babies are quickly chilled. Stay calm and peaceful, even though this is very exciting. Breathe with a gentle expiration as slowly as you comfortably can. You are breathing for your babies.

Once in the second stage, take it as gently as possible and avoid both hyperventilating and prolonged breath holding. Your first baby may cope well with these, but the second baby needs good oxygenation for a while longer. Choose any position that is comfortable for you – preferably an upright one (standing, squatting, kneeling, or half-kneeling, half-squatting). If labor is progressing very rapidly, get on all fours. When the first baby is born, put her to your breast. The sucking will stimulate further contractions to bring the next baby to birth.

## The Baby Who Is Slow To Breathe

Babies are enormously adaptable. Then can manage with very little oxygen for much longer than an adult. Some babies start to breathe as soon as their heads are born. Most take a few seconds to get going. When the cord is not clamped immediately, and it is pulsating, the baby is still receiving oxygenated blood straight into her bloodstream. There need be no rush to force her to breathe.

When a baby is born with the mother in an upright position mucus drains naturally from the mouth and nose. Newborn babies often sneeze mucus out very effectively too. If a baby needs help to breathe, the first thing to do is to make sure that the airways are clear. She can be placed on her front with the head lower than the hips, so that mucus drains out, while you gently massage her back. If your baby has had a long and difficult transition she will need warmth most of all. Otherwise she uses up a great deal of energy trying to maintain body heat. Most heat loss is from the head, so she should be wrapped in warmed flannel blankets and her head covered.

There can be a spiritual element in helping a baby to life. If your baby is just flickering and is starting, but not quite managing, to breathe, it helps to talk to your baby, to say "Hello, baby," "Come on love, come on!" or "You're beautiful!" The result may be that the lungs open wider, breaths are deeper, and respiration is more regular. In intensive care nurseries, where babies are being monitored very carefully, oxygen levels often rise when a baby is stroked and when the mother speaks to her baby.

## You Have Heavy Bleeding

During your pregnancy a steady flow of blood or continual spotting can mean that the placenta is starting to peel away from the lining of the uterus (placental abruption) or that it is in front of the baby's head (placenta previa). Let your midwife or doctor know what is happening. They will probably get you into hospital as quickly as they can, as an examination should only be done once everything has been set up for cesarean section, should it be necessary.

After your labor and delivery your uterus continues to contract, although you may not be aware of it. The placenta cannot contract, so it peels away from the lining of the uterus, usually within half an hour of the birth, and slips down into your vagina. When this happens and the placenta is ready to be expelled, some bright red blood appears and the cord lengthens. Until the placenta separates from the uterine wall there is no bleeding and even though the placenta may remain in the uterus for a long time, this is not dangerous. Your midwife or doctor may gently press in above your pubic bone and push upward toward your navel to see if the cord moves up as the uterus is tipped upward. If it does, the placenta is still attached and no one should pull on the cord or it may cause bleeding.

The best way to assist your body in detaching from your placenta is to stand upright and blow into an empty bottle. As air is exhaled, the abdominal press comes into play so that the mother's abdominal muscles press on her fundus and propel the placenta down. Tugging or pulling on the cord can cause hemorrhage and should never be done. A postpartum hemorrhage happens when a placenta does not peel away completely, and blood seeps from gaping sinuses in the muscle wall of the uterus. Left to itself the uterus will clamp down uniformly and will sheer off the placenta in one smooth sweep, but if poked and prodded may only release in certain sections.

Gently massaging your uterus and nipple stimulation will keep your uterus firm and contracting to assist in the birth of your placenta. When the placenta is delivered, your midwife or doctor will check your pulse and blood pressure and may ask you to continue massaging the uterus to keep it well contracted.

## Home Birth Advantages

A carefully planned and lovingly conducted home birth, in which the rhythms of nature are respected and the woman is nurtured by attendants who have the knowledge and understanding to support the spontaneous unfolding of life, is the safest kind of birth there is, and the most deeply satisfying for everyone involved."

Reprinted with kind permission from, Homebirth – The Essential Guide to Giving Birth Outside of the Hospital, Sheila Kitzinger. A practical, fact-filled guide for every woman who wants to choose carefully among the alternatives to giving birth in a hospital by the leading female authority on pregnancy and childbirth. Further work by Sheila Kitzinger includes The Politics of Birth, The New Experience of Childbirth, The New Pregnancy and Childbirth - Choices and Challenges, Birth Your Way, Rediscovering Birth, Becoming a Grandmother, and Birth Over Thirty Five. You can find out more about her work at www.sheilakitzinger.com.

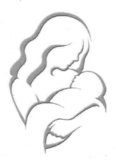

# Chapter 10 - Your Partner's Role in Childbirth

More men than ever, to their credit, are taking an active, involved interest in the birth of their children. Your partner wants to be involved by becoming a part of the decision process. Your partner has a critical role to play as your advocate. Write your birth plan together so that everyone is aware of what is important to you.

Your partner is not professional labor support unless your partner has personally birthed a baby. Fathers are "birthing" as well and this situation is just as new to him as it is to you. Hiring professional labor support, such as a doula or midwife, during your first birth is an excellent investment and can take the pressure off your partner. Your partner and family can then provide the emotional support that is just as necessary.

Make sure you have a partner. Your partner does not have to be your mate; anyone you love and trust will do.

Your birth partner, whether your mate, your midwife, your mother, your sister, your best friend, your next door neighbor, or a combination of the above will give you the emotional support necessary to see you through.

The support of your partner will often depend on the preparation they have received in prenatal classes. The Bradley Method of Husband-Coached Childbirth classes focus on giving your partner adequate knowledge so that they can become your advocate in labor.

You may wish to have people you know come in shifts if you have a large family or many supportive friends. Having a few people come in on and off during your labor can help you to keep your sense of humor when you need it most. Birth is a great celebration of life and touches deeply all involved in the process.

Here are a few ideas of what your partner can do for you during labor and delivery:

- Ask your partner to make sure that you have plenty of water, juices and tea to drink.
- Have your partner remind you to breathe slowly and deeply.
- Have your partner remind you to urinate every hour to make more room for your baby's descent.
- Have your partner massage your lower back, neck and shoulders. Current research shows that as you become more relaxed during labor your pain decreases. Thus a warm bath or shower, a gentle massage, a shoulder to lean against, a gentle hug, encouraging words and a hand to grip will aid greatly in naturally reducing pain during labor.
- Let your partner know before labor how much you love him. Warn him that sometimes women say things during labor that they don't mean. Let him know not to take anything personally.
- Your partner is your cheering section. Even whispered words of encouragement can help see you through to the end.
- Be clear in telling your partner what you need during labor, don't assume or expect your partner will know what you want during each stage.
- Walk around the hospital as much as possible during your labor and use your partner to lean on during contractions. Having someone to lean on when you are standing during a contraction seems to shorten the length of the contraction.
- Your partner should encourage you to change positions whenever you can. Moving into a new position, standing, walking, resting on the left side, kneeling, moving to the bath, climbing stairs, squatting, and leaning over furniture helps your body and your baby to work more efficiently.
- During delivery, have your partner hold the mirror so that you can see your baby's head crown to more easily control the pushing stage.
- Have your partner or professional labor support use the warmed oil you have brought to massage your perineum and your baby's head to ease delivery.
- Have your partner or professional labor support provide gentle counter pressure to your baby's head and your perineum allowing for a safe, controlled delivery of the shoulders and chest.
- Have your partner or midwife bring your baby to your breast for the first time as quickly as possible after birth. Breastfeeding immediately after birth releases hormones to help your body birth the placenta and to stop excessive bleeding.

- Standing while blowing into an empty bottle will also help your body to more efficiently release your placenta. Never let anyone pull on the cord of your placenta. This can cause bleeding. There is no hurry for the placenta to be delivered or removed.
- Have your partner be in charge of cutting your baby's umbilical cord. Some couples tie the umbilical cord with a cotton cord instead using of a plastic clamp. The umbilical cord seems to heal faster with less chance of infection when cotton is used.
- Ask your partner to closely examine the placenta. Look at your placenta as well to assure yourself that the entire placenta has been delivered.
- Have your partner take your baby's first pictures using the disposable instant flash camera you have brought along. Disposable cameras are easy to work, always ready and allow you to be sure you will capture the first precious moments of your baby's life.
- Invite your professional labor support person to take your first family photograph of the three of you together. You will always treasure these photographs.

## What You Need to Know before You Have Your Baby: Professional Labor Support – What to Expect

### Early First Stage of Childbirth – Prelabor & Labor

"The efforts of the doula or childbirth assistant during the first stage, when the cervix thins and opens, should be geared toward helping the mother have a relaxed body and a mind at peace. This allows the mother's contracting uterus to open her cervix while she conserves her energy for pushing. You can help her with the following measures:

Have the mother stay home as long as possible. Options for comfort are much greater at home. Going into the hospital will not make things happen faster, and labor may even slow down in a strange environment.

During this early time in labor a woman can gradually get used to the feeling of contractions. Later, as contractions become more intense, they will hurt. This pain is a normal part of the birthing process. Remind the mother that there is a purpose for the pain; it is a sign of the work her body is doing to thin and open her cervix. To help her accept and cope with the pain, you can remind her that she is not in this alone.

It is essential for a woman to take nourishment in the form of fluids or easily digestible proteins and carbohydrates. A dehydrated or starved body cannot labor as effectively as a well nourished one. Also, the baby continues to be totally dependent on her for nourishment throughout labor. Suggest that she eat a good meal early in labor, and have her continue to drink plenty of liquids and avoid high-fat foods and concentrated sweets. The mother might wish to try juice, fruit, yogurt, whole-wheat bread or crackers, nourishing soup, and other foods that appeal to her. As labor progresses, she may not feel like eating, but encourage her to drink. Labor is hard work, and she will need lots of fluid to meet her body's needs. If fruit juices do not appeal to her, suggest non-caffeinated soft drinks, which will give her the energy she needs without making her feel jittery. Nausea is normal for some women in labor and is not the result of drinking or eating.

Suggest a warm bath to help her stay more comfortable and relaxed. Fill the tub as high as possible. Have her kneel in the tub or lie back against pillows. Keep a comfortably hot, wet towel over her belly and groin during contractions. She might want a cool drink and a cool cloth for her head. Be sure to give this a try, especially at times in labor when the mother feels that nothing will help.

Have the mother walk. Walking tends to shorten labor, reduce the need for pain-relieving drugs, decrease fetal heart-rate abnormalities, and improve the baby's condition during labor and birth. A doula and other support people may need to keep encouraging the mother strongly to walk.

Women in labor should change positions often-at least every thirty to sixty minutes. This can help to avoid or correct fetal distress, as well as speed labor. Positions such as standing, squatting, and kneeling while leaning forward are excellent. They can increase uterine activity, shorten labor by helping the cervix dilate more efficiently, and reduce discomfort. Other good positions for labor include sitting, lying on the side, and being up on the hands and knees. Use lots of pillows to help the mother feel comfortable. She should not lie flat on her back because this can cause a drop in her blood pressure and a decreased blood flow and therefore decrease the oxygen to her baby. Laboring women should urinate every hour. A full bladder can inhibit uterine activity and be an obstacle to the baby's birth.

## Late First Stage of Childbirth – Transition Period

During the late first stage of labor, most women strongly need other people, their support people, to help them cope with and accept the intense contractions that are normal for this time in labor. Labor is truly easier when a woman has people to encourage and reassure her during this time. If she is going to a hospital or birth center for her baby's birth, the best time to make the trip is usually late in the first stage. Whether at home or in the hospital or birth center, the following measures will continue to be helpful:

Have the mother continue with warm baths or showers, hot towels, position changes, walking, nourishment, and frequent urination. Try other comfort measures such as cold compresses, pressure on her back, pelvic rocking, massages or stroking. Let the mother use extra pillows, a bean bag, you or the father to lean against for added comfort. What feels good often changes as labor progresses, so remember to try again with comfort measures that may not have been helpful earlier.

This is an intense time. The mother may need to maintain contact with you through every contraction. You can talk and breathe her through contractions, use a loving touch, and maintain eye contact. Then help her rest, relax and refresh herself between contractions. Visualizations and imagery are also extremely useful to help the mother work through the contractions.

Ask the mother to show or tell you not only how and where to touch her but also what feels good and what does not.

Help the mother stay upright and walking as long as possible. Alternate periods of activity and rest as needed. She may need a lot of encouragement to change position, walk, or urinate. Remember, these activities will help her labor progress normally.

Many women experience a time in labor when they are in a lot of pain and cannot get comfortable. If the mother experiences these feelings, help her concentrate on releasing tension and yielding to the intense contractions. Emotional support and focus on relaxation, in spite of the intensity of the contractions, will get her through this difficult time. Reassure her that she can do it. Have her deal with her contractions one at a time and not think about how long it has been or how long it will be.

## The Second Stage of Childbirth – Delivery

The doula's efforts and those of the father during the second stage, when the cervix is completely open and the mother pushes her baby out, should be geared not only toward helping her cooperate with her body but also toward providing a calm, peaceful atmosphere into which her new child will be born.

During this stage you, the doula, can help in the following ways: There is nothing magical about a woman being at ten centimeters, or completely dilated. Some women feel an urge to push before ten centimeters, and others feel it considerably after this point.

If the mother does not feel an urge to push, try getting her into a gravity assisted upright position and continue to breathe with her through contractions. Walking, squatting, or sitting on the toilet often helps at this time. Remind the mother to be patient, relax, and wait for a pushing urge to develop as her baby moves farther down her birth canal. Waiting until the urge to push develops allows her to coordinate her pushing efforts with those of her uterus. If her physician or midwife feels it is necessary to birth her baby quickly, she or he will direct her on how and when to push.

Have the woman urinate before she begins pushing.

Any positions used for labor can also be used for pushing and for the baby's birth. Each position has advantages and disadvantages. A mother who has practiced during pregnancy and experimented during labor may know the most comfortable and effective positions. Help her change positions at least every half hour if she has a long or difficult second stage.

Upright positions that use gravity may be helpful. Squatting uses gravity and allows maximum opening of the pelvic outlet. Standing sometimes helps if the baby is still high in the pelvis. Sitting on the toilet is excellent for opening up and releasing the whole pelvic area. Lying on one side can be helpful in slowing a quick descent, but less helpful if the baby is coming slowly. Upright positions can aggravate hemorrhoids; lying on the side does not.

All fours positions do not use gravity, but they do take pressure off the back and allow spreading of the hips and pelvic bones. Both all fours and squatting positions are good for a large or posterior baby.

Avoid letting the mother lie flat on her back. If she is semi-reclining, you or the father can sit behind her to prop her up, or you can use pillows or raise the head of the birthing bed or delivery table so that she is not lying flat.

The mother will need frequent assurance that the intense and painful sensations she may feel – backache, nausea, hot flashes, trembling legs, spreading sensations in the pelvis, intense pressure on the rectum, an urge to empty the bowels, involuntary bearing down, intense pressure as the baby descends through the birth canal, or burning and stretching sensations as the vaginal outlet opens to accommodate her baby – are normal and that she can stretch and open enough to give birth to her baby.

Remind her to work with her body – let her body tell her what to do to get her baby out. She can bear down, push, when, how, and however long her body demands that. Encourage her to ease up on pushing if it hurts or if burning sensations occur. She may want to see and touch her baby's head as it emerges from her body. This contact may renew her spirits and energy, and help her focus on bringing her baby out.

When pushing, she might at times breathe out, make noise, or hold her breath. Many women have found that certain noises like grunts and moaning sounds help them give birth to their babies. Help her not to be inhibited about making sounds which is a natural part of the birthing process for many women, and she will find what works for her if she goes ahead and tries it. Many women find that releasing sound opens the throat and subsequently the birth canal. Have her avoid prolonged breath holding.

During a long second stage, a woman needs nourishment to keep up or restore her energy level. Spoonfuls of honey or drinks sweetened with honey or juice will provide a quick source of energy.

You can encourage her to release and open for the birth. If you watch her mouth, shoulders, and legs for signs of tension, you can help her release these areas. She may be so intently focused on the work of giving birth that she does not hear what others are saying. You can help by keeping the mother informed of what is happening and conveying instructions from the health team or midwife.

Keep the atmosphere calm and peaceful, so that the mother and father can enjoy the end of labor and the new life they have brought forth."

Reprinted with kind permission from Mothering the Mother – How A Doula Can Help You Have a Shorter, Easier, and Healthier Birth Marshall H Klaus, M.D., John H. Kennell, M.D., and Phyllis H. Klaus, M.Ed.,C.S.W.

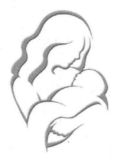

# Chapter 11 - Secrets to Having a Safe and Gentle Labor and Delivery

## Labor

- Labor contractions are very similar to your period cramps when they begin.
- Your labor can take days or hours.
- Hire professional labor support to assist you and your partner.
- Practice, pre-pack and pre-plan for this special day.
- Remain as "relaxed" and as focused as you can.
- Work with your body.
- Trust yourself and your body to deliver your baby safely.
- Breath deeply throughout your labor. Your baby and your body need all the oxygen you can give now. See yourself giving your baby extra energy with each long slow breath you take. Work together with your baby and see your baby beginning to descend out through your birth canal as your cervix slowly and easily expands to allow your baby's head through.
- Remember that each contraction brings you one step closer to your baby's birth.
- Visualize your cervix dilating as two great oak doors sliding slowly open. Or as a rose gently opening its petals.
- Don't be embarrassed during your labor, the doctors, nurses and midwives have seen it all. Modesty can inhibit your labor, save it for after your baby is born.
- If anyone is upsetting you with their presence during your labor feel free to ask them to leave the room.
- Focus on having your body work with the contraction. Feel your cervix opening with each contraction and visualize your baby moving further

down towards the opening. Working with the contractions and surrendering to them will help to move your baby along.

- Don't waste your energy and your body's oxygen supply by screaming or fighting. Your energy is the fuel needed to propel your baby into the world. Anything else is counterproductive.
- Grunting or groaning at a low level can help when you feel intense pain.
- Your mind can be your most powerful resource during childbirth. Use your mind to focus inward on the rhythm of your labor.
- Take an epidural only as a last resort. An epidural can cause serious side effects to you and your baby, as well as slow down the most critical part of your labor. The greatest stress on your body happens during the transition stage of your labor and an epidural will not work at this stage.
- During labor walk and stand as much as possible. Gravity will help your baby through your birth canal. Placing your arms around your partner and slightly suspending your weight on him can lessen the pain of a contraction and will assist in moving your baby down.
- Moving about during your labor will help you to feel more in control and will make your labor faster and easier. Change your position as often as you can. Go from sitting or standing, to sitting on the toilet, to leaning forward on the bed, to a squatting position on the floor, to a rocking chair, walking up or down stairs, back to the shower and back again to the toilet.
- If you are experiencing back labor moving to all fours either on the floor or bed will help your team to work on massaging your back to ease muscle spasms. A warm shower or bath is also an excellent way to reduce the pain of back labor. Counter pressure applied during contractions to your tailbone can help as well.
- Holding your partner's hand can give you the extra strength you need at this time.
- Try putting your focus on a favorite photograph or favorite song.
- Fighting and tensing up will increase the pain. Accepting, relaxing and working with the wave-like contractions will decrease the pain.

## Delivery

- Delivery feels very similar to having a bowel movement.
- Delivery can last hours or minutes.
- Reach down and feel your baby's head with your hand to connect with the miracle of your baby's birth.

- Touching your baby as the head crowns can also help you to focus your energy.
- Squatting opens your pelvic area by 30% and speeds delivery.
- Sitting on the toilet is a good birthing position as it is one of the best ways to isolate the muscles you will use to push your baby out.
- A squatting bar on the bed is also an excellent birthing position as it allows you total control and you can view your baby's head crowning in a mirror.
- Plan to have your perineum massaged with warm oil as this will stretch the muscles and help your baby to slide out easily. Warm water compresses can also help the perineum to stretch without tearing.
- Squatting for the final stages of delivery can help you to retain some sense of privacy.
- When pushing, use your vaginal muscles to keep your baby from moving back from the birth opening at the end of the contraction. Short pushes are much more effective than long strenuous pushing. Continue even breathing. Short pants with your pushes can be very effective. Watching in the mirror will help you to isolate these muscles more easily.
- When asked to stop pushing, make sure you do. An extra push at this time can cause you to tear. The easiest delivery for both baby and mother is a slow, controlled delivery. Remind yourself that the pain will end the moment your baby is fully born.
- The "ring of fire", as your baby's head crowns fully, is the most painful part of childbirth. Luckily nature is kind and with an unmedicated birth crowning rarely lasts for longer than three pushes.
- Proper perineum support from your professional labor coach will also help to create a slow, controlled delivery.
- If you are told to stop pushing and are having difficulty with it, switch to a kneeling position and you will have more control.
- Should any difficulty arise during your delivery your best position will be in a supported squat, allowing your baby every bit of extra room needed for a faster delivery.
- Put your baby immediately to your breast, within moments after birth. In your baby's first hour the natural instinct to suck is the strongest. Most babies know how to suck, just make your breast available. Do not let your baby suck on just your nipple, make sure your baby's mouth is open wide enough to allow the entire areola, or most of it, as well as your nipple into the mouth as this is the correct latch. Breastfeed as long as you feel

comfortable on each side. Always express some drops of milk or colostrum and let air dry on your nipple after feeding to heal any nipple soreness. Do not take breastfeeding advice from anyone who has never breastfed. Professional female assistance is needed for all matters concerning breastfeeding.

- As you are breastfeeding your baby for the first time, oxytocin will be naturally released throughout your system to help your body to slow down blood loss and to eject your placenta. You will feel more contractions now as your body works to expel your placenta.

- Stand and blow into an empty bottle to assist your body to expel your placenta.

- Do not allow anyone to tug or pull on the cord for your placenta. Allow your body to slowly release your placenta. There is no reason for this stage to be rushed.

- Have your partner check your placenta once it is delivered for any missing pieces or sections. This is the most critical aspect of having a safe birth and delivery. If any of the placenta is left inside of your womb, it can lead to you being unable to bear any more children. Ask to see the placenta yourself to assure yourself that it has been completely delivered.

- Have your partner feed you right after delivery and it will bring your energy up again.

- Plan to Kangaroo Care your baby for the first week. Keeping your baby in bed with you and constantly at your side during this time will increase your baby's immunity and help you to feel more attached to your baby.

- If you are in a hospital and you feel well you may want to take your baby home with you in the next few hours and have your health team come into your home to check on you and your new baby in the days to follow. If you choose a free-standing birth clinic you will naturally be leaving with your baby in two or three hours with the midwives coming to your home for each of the next three days.

## What You Need To Know Before You Have Your Baby: Why Do We Need A Gentle Beginning?

"Human birth is the most miraculous, transformational, and mysterious event of our lives. It is an event shared by every single member of the human race. The birth experience imprints itself indelibly upon the lives of the mother and the baby she is bringing forth.

In recent centuries, humans began to explore and experiment with science and the development of high technology. A combination of natural human characteristics such as curiosity, a desire to control, fear of that which seems beyond human control, and concentrated focus upon the application of technology, has crept into and diverted cultural perspective and respect for the sacredness of the birth experience. The result of this technological focus and experimentation is apparent within the dominant cultures, in the form of entire populations sharing high levels of stress, fear, and emotional dysfunction.

The Industrial Revolution in America accelerated a trend for exploration in managing birth. Lifestyles changed, cities became quickly crowded without immediate understanding of disease control. Maternal and infant mortality rates climbed and hospitals were erroneously seen as a new and safer place for all to give birth, rather than homes. Driven by the competition of the free market, a strong emphasis was placed on themes of independence. It was believed that fostering close emotional ties between mothers and babies would foster dependency, and unproductive people. John Watson, a well known behaviorist in his time, led a convincing campaign for teaching new parenting theory, suited to American progress in the late 1920's. He strongly discouraged holding babies, kissing or touching babies or children. He encouraged parents to ignore the cries of their babies in order to regiment sleep and feeding schedules, and in order to prevent mothers from becoming "slaves" to demanding children forever.

Western culture has begun to acknowledge that this way of parenting is not ideal. Slowly, we are beginning to recognize the severe consequences of such practices. Scientific research on brain development is leading us back to the realization that we have been blind to essential components of birth which profoundly influence the entire lifetime of those involved. A branch of anthropologic study, now termed ethnopediatrics, has also noted through close to a century of cross - cultural research, that the well being of mothers and their babies reflects the core health and function of the community in general. Mothers and their babies, supported in their early adjustment, bonding and breastfeeding, provide the community with reliable, emotionally secure and productive participants, benefiting all. Westernized culture lost sight of this critical information with the advent of Industrialization. Interestingly, science has begun to rediscover this ancient wisdom, and science is currently the voice most often heard.

Birth, like death, is an innate part of life, unique to the individual, and in most cases does not require the medical interventions and control we have been told is necessary. It is high illusion to imagine that we, as humans, can control this process. To instead show deep respect, awe, and trusting surrender is more appropriate and in alignment with this amazing rite of passage.

## Philosophy of Gentle Birth

Gentle Birth does not dictate a list of rules that must be followed. It is an approach to birth that incorporates a woman's individual values and beliefs. Every birth is a powerful experience – sometimes painful, always transformational. Each birth is as unique as the mother and baby experiencing it.

The elements that make up a gentle birth are certainly nothing new or revolutionary. Many have been a part of childbirth for thousands of years. A gentle birth relies on the understanding that labor is a part of a mysterious continuum of physiological events, beginning with conception and continuing well into the first years of life. Mother and baby, inseparable and interdependent, work together as a unit from the fertilization of the egg until weaning from breastfeeding takes place. The resulting bonds created during this period are foundational within those lives.

Pregnancy provides a woman with valuable and heightened awareness of the intangible aspects of herself and of life. Support in accessing her innate wisdom, guidance with education, and modeling of trust, allows her to more easily release previously learned resistance or fear. This facilitates a Gentle Birth experience.

> Nature is already as good as it can be
> It cannot be improved upon
> He who tries to redesign it, spoils it
> He who tries to redirect it, misleads it
> > -Lao-tzu

## Vision

To recognize, embrace, support the optimal opportunity for a gentle, healthy beginning in life is one of the most intimate, simple and globally healing efforts anyone can engage in. As more people rediscover, appreciate, and implement this approach to entry into life, we can expect that the emerging generation, and generations thereafter will enjoy greater connection to well being as the order of the universe. The prospect of activating and perpetuating increased levels of well being for all can be a source of current inspiration, hope and well being for those who begin to embark on this path. Everyone can benefit.

## Essence of a Gentle Birth

A gentle birth takes place when a woman is supported by the people she chooses to be with during this most intimate time. She needs to be loved and nurtured by those around her so she can feel comfortable and secure enough to follow her natural instincts. During a natural, gentle birth a woman feels and senses the power of the birth and uses this energy to transform every part of her own being. A gentle birth is not rushed. The baby emerges at its own pace and in its own time. It is received into the hands of those who love and recognize it as a human being with its own life purpose, only beginning to unfold. Following are suggestions for assisting women to create their own gentle experience.

## Key Elements:

### *Preparation*

Throughout history women learned to give birth intuitively. They watched their mothers, family members and others in the community give birth as they grew from children to women, ready to carry on the reproductive cycle of life. Familiarity eliminated unnecessary fears and anxieties. They engaged in cultural rituals and information sharing as well as observing and feeling the indescribable. This created a well-rounded inspiring education, ideal for nurturing a spirit/ mind/ body connection.

Due to many decades of technologic experimentation, several generations of mothers in America lost an opportunity to learn about birth intuitively. Indeed, in conjunction with the emergence of the medical establishment, and their discrediting of the value of midwifery, attitudes toward birth changed dramatically. A radical and misguided priority began to govern the treatment of women experiencing reproductive activity. The priorities focused upon creating independent individuals who were driven to thrive in the free market economy. A life embracing perspective had been abandoned in favor of treating symptoms as they appeared, with science being called upon as the only valid method for problem solving in a progressive world. Birth began to be viewed as pathology, and the medical community came to view themselves as able and responsible for controlling and modifying all pathology.

Extensive use of anesthesia, routine and unnecessary interventions, isolation of laboring mothers and separation of mothers and babies, became associated with safe and modern practices. Parents were encouraged to resist showing affection for their children, and directed to show caring through methods which excluded physical touch and contact. Massive and persistent campaigns undermined trust in the body, and promoted transferring all trust to the ultimate authority of the day, physicians. Many American mothers and grandmothers have little memory of any birth experience. By 1955, 95 percent of all American births took place in a hospital with an alluring and fashionable objective of painless and safe birth through anesthesia. When women became coerced into desiring painless birth, they also relinquished their own power to the medical technicians and physicians. Those women who have vague memories of their hospital experiences often tell stories of humiliation, frustration and disempowerment. The concept of joyful birth often seems alien to them as they hear of the changes taking place in recent years. They are amazed to watch their grandchildren begin to view birth differently, from an increasingly empowered perspective. Childbirth educators are needed now to recreate the knowledge previously learned intuitively and through one's own mother or family, to engender current and future generations with the previously lost vital connection to birth.

Educators can help expectant mothers learn about the life process, the design of labor and birth, and how to best nurture good health and a positive and hopeful attitude. They can show pregnant mothers varieties of coping techniques and encourage them to empower themselves by trusting their own choices and preferences. Educators can show families how to access resources gaining useful information and the knowledge of available alternatives. Educators can provide a theoretical "new image" mirror to hold up to an expectant mother and point out what has always been there but not previously noticed. Educators can encourage women to internally assess how she feels about her sexuality, her relationship with the father, her relationship with her own parents and any other beliefs surrounding birth which she might hold.

When a pregnant mother encounters supportive, informed guidance, she will be able to develop self esteem and confidence. When a pregnant mother has had time to prepare herself emotionally, it will be easier for her to surrender any resistance in her birthing process. Previously confusing topics will become clearer for her. She will be able to more clearly define her own preferences within this context. This will lead to planning, greater understanding and a feeling of preparation. Preparation replaces anxiety and fear with focus, direction and greater calm. Research has clearly demonstrated that childbirth education has a powerful and beneficial influence upon the unfolding of a laboring experience and birth.

## A Reassuring Environment

A laboring woman has 8 times more oxytocin receptors occurring in her body than at any other time in her life. This combined with endorphins, provides her with a natural aid to enhance her labor and bonding experience. When she is comfortable, distraction-free, and believes herself to be in a safe environment, she is able to access the primal nature of her hindbrain, which will lead her through the process. Laboring and birth are a parasympathetic experience. Comparatively, the sympathetic experience is associated with the "fight or flight" response and increased catecholamine production. Catecholamines such as epinephrine and norepinephrine, will both undermine the effects of and stop production of the oxytocin and endorphins needed to help with labor.

In the parasympathetic mode, the dark, quiet environment will help a woman to feel safe and to access her instinctive nature more easily. She will tend to conserve energy more efficiently, influencing the duration of her labor. For her to be soothed during and between contractions, in whatever way appeals to her, will allow her to maintain this complex physiologic state. This in turn will be conveyed to the infant during the labor as well as at birth. The infant relies on its mother's reactions to labor and birth as an indicator of its own safety. Even in a case where a mother chooses to labor vocally and with loud sounds, the infant can still sense the difference between a mother having chosen to follow her instinctual pattern and a mother who is panicky and afraid. That mother and baby are a team, working through this transformation together, by intention, reduces infant stress and allows for easier bonding and normal physiologic process.

Additionally, the assignment of each unique birth to a standardized arbitrary schedule is antithetical to the process, undermines trust, and creates stress in a laboring woman, pulling her out of her hind brain to try to function in a mode which does not serve her as well.

Using Maslow's Hierarchy of Needs we have a simple template from which to understand and remember the importance of support for a laboring woman and new mother.

The pyramid is divided into 5 spaces horizontally. At the base of the triangle is the core element of physiologic needs. This translates to assuring that mother is rested, fed, hydrated, and in a comfortable temperature environment.

The next space is assigned the category of safety and security. Here we provide the reassuring environment, so she need not worry about her safety, and can allow herself to focus completely upon the laboring process.

The next category addresses love and belonging. Being surrounded by people who care and who love her, facilitates the production of hormones needed to progress.

The top remaining categories are next, self esteem, the confidence gained with help in the three previous categories, and at the top, self actualization, the achievement of her goal, having the entirety of a supportive foundation beneath her.

## Freedom of Movement

A pervasive myth, centuries old but more actively perpetuated in recent decades, is that a laboring mother should be in bed. Restriction of a laboring woman's freedom of movement during labor is not conducive to progress at all. Women need to be able to choose every position they get into as a direct response to subtle instinctive communication between she and her infant during labor and birth. Just as a woman will get an urge to eat or to sleep, she will get urges to take certain positions which will bring her better comfort and coincidentally allow the baby to reposition itself as it moves down and out. Baby will tend to take the path of least resistance in its rotation down and out. It is important for mother to put as little continuous pressure on the moveable portions of pelvis (such as laying continuously in bed) as possible so that baby has opportunity to position optimally for birth. Further, gravity can be a wonderful advantage in bringing baby down.

In addition to allowing optimal space for baby to move down and through the pelvis, freedom of movement also allows for better maternal circulation, which will help her muscles work more efficiently. Freedom of movement also is effective as a coping technique, thus tending to enhance maternal perception of empowerment.

## Quiet

A hushed and quiet atmosphere for laboring can be helpful in reducing infant stress as it goes through the journey of birth. It supports the parasympathetic state of instinctual coping and processing. For those attending to mother, quiet conveys a gentle respect for the intricate interaction of hormones which help to progress labor and also facilitate bonding for mother and baby. Quiet also maintains gentle regard for the heightened sensitivity and sensorial invasion a newborn encounters once born. Even if a mother chooses to make her own higher volume sounds, if she is purposely choosing to express, and chooses tones in the lower octaves rather than high, the baby will sense that she is not panicked.

## Low Light

Another key to maintaining the calm of parasympathetic state is low lighting. Newborns have been primarily in the dark during gestation. During the birth process, low light provides the most comfortable environment for mother and child. Low light creates a relaxing and private atmosphere in which a special, intimate event can take place. A room lit with natural light, candles, or very low wattage electric light provides an ideal ambience for a laboring woman. After the birth, the child's eyes are spared from bright lights. The most amazing thing has been witnessed in darkened birthing rooms: Newborn babies almost immediately open their eyes and begin to gaze at their mothers. Gazing into the eyes of your newly emerged child, who seems peaceful and present, is an unforgettable moment.

## Continuous Labor Support

The benefits of an experienced, caring, supportive person whom the mother trusts, have now been well documented by Dr. Marshall Klaus and his co-researchers. In their scientific study they were able to determine that the difference in labor outcome, between mother being alone, and mother being supported, was highly significant. In the three control groups, the mothers who were left alone to labor had the most incidence of poor outcome, and of negative perception of the labor and birth experience. Mothers with a person sitting in the room continuously, without otherwise interacting, had much better outcomes and perceptions. The mothers who were given continuous interactive labor support showed the highest statistical difference in outcome and perception. These mothers had 50% fewer surgical births, requested painkilling medication 60% less often than the others, and also had much lower incidence of interventions such as forceps or vacuum deliveries.

Regardless of the amount of intellectual training a woman has, the intensity of labor, and the newness of physiologic responses she likely never before encountered will tend to surprise her and shake her confidence. It is at those moments, that the loving care of a trusted companion or several, will be most appreciated. Their reassurance that all is well and progressing, the physical care they can provide, and reflection to her of the marvel of how she is coping will be useful.

## Labor Starts on Its Own

Nature has always had its own pace and series of cycles. In all living things, there is a time of increase and a time of decrease. A time of growing, a peak, and a decline, even as a cycle within a larger cycle. Fruit ripens and falls from a tree. Trees shed their leaves and have new growth. It is logical to trust that the design of a healthy human gestation follows the same principles. Prior to the time when technology and pharmaceuticals were so pervasively used in birth, healthy babies came when the critical balance of complex processes reached a point which initiated labor. They gestate as long as they need to and then come into the world.

The well known unfolding of events such as head engagement, preparatory contractions, a softening cervix, greater maternal hip joint laxity, to name a few, during the final weeks of pregnancy illustrate the wisdom of biologic design. Despite extensive research and technology, there remains deep mystery surrounding exactly what takes place in this process. It is still difficult to determine the moment of conception definitively, and still difficult to predetermine the perfect moment when labor will start. The methods used for determining due dates are more accurately termed "educated approximations" based upon usually incomplete information. Only 15% of women have a 28 day menstrual cycle, yet the conventional methods in use today are based upon an assumption of a 28 day cycle. Therefore, an induction of labor is based upon considerable guesswork. Induction as a common occurrence (36%) in America, has created ample opportunities for research. This research has shown us that to artificially initiate labor for any but the most critical medical reasons, is to create an unnecessary and potentially serious risk to mother and baby.

### The First Breath

At the moment a child takes its first breath, fetal circulation is quickly altered to infant circulation. While the changing values will be effective in a healthy newborn, it takes time for them to adjust to this new way of existence. It will take time for the new pathways to become permanent. The newborn must adjust to breathing at a different rate, heart rate slowing slightly, and it must adjust to the multitude of powerful new sensations it is encountering, including the sensation of cold air entering its lungs.

A gentle birth supports the new found discovery that normal newborns do not need immediate invasive suctioning and vigorous wiping and rubbing to begin breathing. These practices, as protocols, can be scary to the newborn. The newborn senses there is fear behind those practices, a sense of urgency, a fear of losing control, fear of the loss of life if immediate aggressive action is not taken. These attitudes, however well intended, do not convey the needed sense of welcoming and are not at all gentle.

### The First Caresses

An unhurried and undisturbed interaction between mother and baby is one of the most pinnacle moments in the new life of the child. The feel of skin to skin contact, being held, soothed, welcomed have a powerful calming effect on the newborn. Touching and massaging the newborn is beneficial for both mother and baby. The mothers instinctual reaction is to smell and lightly touch the baby with her fingertips. In a gentle birth the mother is asked to determine the sex of her baby by either looking or feeling under the warm blankets. Within the first few moments of birth the mother's body will experience an enduring bliss which facilitates a flood of emotional bonding, protection and love.

How a baby is received and how it experiences these first few moments of life is utterly important and permanently imprinted upon it's memory. Baby is born with a genetic encoding, a preprogrammed expectation, which activates certain areas of its brain and nervous system as it encounters it's mothers left breast. Mothers throughout all cultures and geographic locations instinctively cradle their babies in this position where the baby is in contact with her heart rhythm.

### The Baby at the Breast

An extension of this wise and ancient biologic design is for the baby to begin sucking on mother's breast within moments after birth. The baby will provide many cues indicating that it is ready to breastfeed when it is born awake and alert with access to its mother. If the baby is not put to the breast within the first hour after birth, she may lapse into a drowsy state that can continue for up to twenty-four hours, making nursing thereafter more difficult. For early nursing to develop easily, the baby's senses must be stimulated to function fully. In a gentle birth, the mother and child are free to communicate with each other without inhibitions.

Not only does this provide increased emotional comfort for the baby, but the stimulation of the mother's nipple causes release of increased oxytocin which will create beneficial uterine contractions. These contractions will work to help expel the placenta and close off blood vessels in the uterus, thus preventing extensive loss of blood. The colostrum extracted by the baby from the breast will populate the infant gastrointestinal tract with beneficial bacteria suited to enhancing digestion, protect the infant with all the antibodies developed by the mother, and provide the infant with a high protein snack. The proximity of the infant to mother when nursing is also a part of the design in that infant vision is clear enough to be able to see his mother's face from this position.

### Bonding and Attachment

One of the most telling examples of the importance of bonding and attachment practices is to look at American culture today reflecting a time when these critical issues were completely misunderstood and overlooked for close to a century. The psychological health of a great many Americans in recent history is in need of much therapy. In a gentle birth the child is not suddenly taken away from her parents to be weighed, measured, and cleaned far from her mother, who is the only safe and familiar person in the world to her. There is no reason or justification for such a practice. In a gentle birth the mother is awake and aware, highly conscious, energized by having given birth, and extremely eager to spend time with her child—touching, feeling, resting or sleeping together. The newborn needs and wants the comforting presence of the mother, her warmth, touch, sound and smell. After a gentle birth most mothers experience an incredible exhilaration that helps them to overcome their exhaustion.

A baby controls himself by attuning to his mother. The mother must be physically present and emotionally available for the baby to be able to interpret where he is in the world. The baby who receives gentle attention and is in attunement with his mother is secure in his knowing, and can more easily trust that his birth has happened for good reasons. The first hours and days after birth are extremely important ones; they can deeply affect the future relationship between mother and parents. Time spent together and alone at this time (and continued through early childhood) will lay the foundation for its entire future of emotional health.

"Wishing you all the best for gentle birth and joy-filled parenting!"

Barbara Harper's expertise in waterbirth and gentle, undisturbed birth is widely sought in all areas of the globe. She has lectured in 36 countries, including many medical, nursing and midwifery programs and universities. Barbara started as a maternity nurse, but went on to become a childbirth educator, doula and midwife. She was always passionate about mothers and babies and learned from an early age what service, sacrifice and hard work were all about, watching her maternal grandmother, who was a nurse and midwife in rural Ohio. Barbara founded Waterbirth International in 1988, after visiting Russia for the first time. Her research and experiences resulted in the publication of Gentle Birth Choices, book and DVD. She also produced Birth Into Being: The Russian Waterbirth Experience in 2000. Midwives and parents alike have called her video programs "the most inspiring birth videos ever produced." Her next book, Embracing the Miracle is in production for release in 2008. Single with three children, Barbara has dedicated her life to helping heal the way we welcome babies into the world. Her two youngest sons were born at home in water. Her daughter was born in a typical 1970s style hospital birth. Barbara resides in Wilsonville, Oregon, a suburb of Portland. There she is active in her church and community and also plays with her grandson, Alex. For more information contact www.waterbirth.org and www.gentlebirthworld.com or call 503-673-0026.

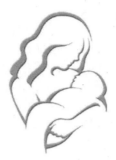

# Chapter 12 - Care of the Mother

- Complete rest during the first few weeks will allow your body to recover quickly and naturally.
- Make a new message for your telephone announcing a new boy or girl, the name of your new baby, and the date and time of birth. Let callers know that you both are resting and you will call back when you can.
- Put a note on the door saying that mom and baby are sleeping and to please call to set up a time to visit.
- Find another new mother for support. Another new mom can help you keep your sense of humor as you begin to adjust to your new roles.
- A calm and quiet environment for both mother and baby for the first thirty days is a custom respected in many tribal societies.
- Take a quick shower or bath every day during the first two weeks. Bring your baby into the bathroom, after a feeding, and lay her down on the bathroom mat if it makes you feel more secure. Your baby will enjoy the noise and steam from the bath and you will appreciate the time to care for yourself.
- Get plenty of rest during the first thirty days. You deserve it. It is easy to feel overwhelmed if you are tired from not getting enough sleep.
- If you feel that you are bleeding excessively, one pad per hour or more, call your doctor immediately.
- If you find a foul odor coming from you, call your doctor immediately.
- In the first few days you may pass larger blood clots. This is normal.
- For hemorrhoids try Vaseline on the affected area between medication applications to avoid irritation.
- You should find your bleeding beginning to taper off and change from bright red, to brown to a light clear discharge after a few weeks. Bed rest is extremely important to help your body to heal itself. If you find yourself

with a bright red discharge all of a sudden, slow down your activities, and bring your baby back to bed with you for two or three days.

- Each time you urinate or change your pad use this opportunity to use a warm water rinse on your vaginal area if you have had an episiotomy. A sports drink bottle with a flip-top can be used to spray warm water as you sit on the toilet. Keep your vaginal area as clean as possible for the first two weeks. Adding Calendula tincture to the warm water rinse can help soothe and heal.

- A light application of Vaseline can also help to soothe an episiotomy area and ease pain upon urination. Clean this away thoroughly afterwards with a warm water rinse.

- Aloe Vera gel can help with itching from an episiotomy site.

- Calendula tincture on pads stored in the freezer can give quick relief from itching at an episiotomy site.

- Arrange to have a sitz bath or Epsom salt bath if episiotomy stitches are bothering you.

- Sleep at every opportunity you find.

- Rest and eat well.

- Set up a half hour or an hour once a day all for yourself. Soak in the tub, read a good book, write a letter to a friend or take the time to balance your checkbook. If your partner is unable to watch your baby for this time, find an older neighbor or hire a young girl for an hour out of each day. It will be just what you need to recharge and appreciate your baby after a break.

- Relax and remember that your baby is new at this too – you are learning together.

- Don't be afraid to ask for help and also to let people know when you've had enough help.

- Ask your caregiver to give most of the baby care over to you, have your caregiver focus on the many other things that need to be done, especially running errands and cooking. Being a parent takes practice, doing the same things over and over and by the second week you will feel much more competent and natural with your new work when you've had this time with your baby.

- You do not have to be overly strong during your home recovery. Ask your doctor for pain relief if necessary.

- If you find cramping a problem as your womb returns to its former size drink raspberry leaf tea, purchased at any health food store, to recondition your uterus. Daily light massage to your lower stomach area can also help to reduce cramping and help to shrink your uterus. Catnip tea can also help with after pains.

- If you have not had a bowel movement in three days you might want to try an enema. An enema will soften your bowel movement so that you are less likely to disturb any surgery site, if you have one.

- Contact a school for massage if you are feeling pain in your neck or shoulders. Many schools allow the students to practice on you at a much reduced price and you can bring your baby along with you. Feed your baby before your appointment and bring your baby into the massage school in your car seat and you will easily have an hour or two of uninterrupted time just for you.

- If you have trouble urinating let your doctor know immediately.

- Make a plan to care for yourself immediately after the first morning feeding for your baby. Your baby will usually be contented and sleepy after the first feeding and you may find this is the only time for personal grooming during the day. Have a shower or bath, put on your make-up if you usually wear it and spend extra time on your hair. When you care for yourself first you will find that you have more to give to your baby.

- Watch out for the "super woman" syndrome. Yes, the cleaning can wait. Take the extra moments in the day to relax, recharge and get to know your new baby. Use shortcuts whenever you can. Leave the laundry in the basket when necessary. Put your feet up whenever you can and have short power naps. Your body has amazing recuperative abilities and allowing yourself to rest frequently will give your body what it needs at this time.

- If you feel overwhelmed with the dependency of your new baby talk to someone who can understand what you are feeling. This may be your husband, your mother, your best friend or your doctor or midwife. These feelings are natural. You are dealing with new routines, exhaustion and hormones. It is important to reassure yourself that most people will feel overwhelmed by a new baby. Knowing that you are not alone and having a support network of other new mothers can do wonders for your self-confidence and your self-esteem.

- Join a weekly parents group to add to the friends you already know. Your single friends won't always understand the depth of commitment needed to care for a baby and build a family. Very few people have 24 hour jobs unless they happen to be a parent. Find another new mother to complain to, be empathetic to, and laugh with as you both experience the joys and challenges of motherhood.

- Continue to take your prenatal vitamins for the first six months after your baby is born, especially if you are breastfeeding. Your body has given a tremendous amount and uses up many of its nutritional stores throughout your pregnancy. By continuing to take your vitamins you will be giving back to your body and creating reserves for the months ahead.

- Choose one day a week or one day a month to reconnect with who you were before. Use this special time to reconnect with your mate, join a dance club, visit single girlfriends, or any favorite activity you have that doesn't scream mommy. This means no scouting out playschools or shopping for baby clothes. A happy mom equals a happy baby. Taking time to be you again will help you to reestablish your equilibrium.

- Take time for yourself, doing things you used to do even if it's only a few minutes here and there because if Mom falls apart, the whole family seems to. Get ready to meet your new body. You may enjoy your new curves but many women feel depressed when their middle section doesn't disappear at once when the baby is delivered. Look into post-natal yoga, mommy and baby exercise classes or deep water workouts. Working out two or three times a week is the best way to pick up your spirits, relieve the stress of your new responsibilities and get you back into your pre-pregnancy shape.

- Your new life will fall into place if you take one step at a time. Get lots of emotional support, accept any offers to help and delegate "duties" if possible to get the rest you deserve and require.

- Recent research from Mothering The New Mother, by Sally Placksin, is showing that postpartum adjustment for a first-time mother realistically takes six months to a year. It takes at least a year to build a working family. Fathers experience the same length of adjustment with a new baby. Create a good support network of other new mothers and families to assist you with enjoying this exciting transition. Many new parents are finding the recent proliferation of parenting classes to be worthwhile and supportive for adapting to the new changes.

# What You Need To Know Before You Have Your Baby: Ten Reasons Why Parents Question Vaccination

"For some time now, members of the government and the medical industry have tried to explain away the phenomenon of parental refusal to vaccinate. Despite the government's own studies, such as Rogers and Pilgrim; 1993, which shows that "Older, highly educated parents form the basis of the [sic] anti-immunization lobby", parents continue to be accused of being ignorant, uncaring and stupid for refusing vaccines which the medical community claim will keep their children healthy.

In an effort to set the record straight, the Australian Vaccination Network, Inc., a national health lobby group and registered charitable organization which is contacted by more than 10,000 Australian parents each year who question this procedure, would like to give you the 10 most common reasons why the parents who contact us have chosen not to vaccinate.

## 1- Vaccines have never been tested.

The gold standard of medical science is the double blind crossover placebo study. This test has never been performed on any vaccine currently licensed in Australia. In an astounding leap of logic, contrary to all rules of science, vaccines are assumed to be safe and effective and therefore, it is considered to be unethical to withhold vaccinations for the purposes of testing them.

## 2- Vaccines contain toxic additives and heavy metals.

The list of vaccine ingredients includes toxins such as formaldehyde, a substance which the Queensland Poisons Control Centre has said was "unsafe at any level if injected into the human body"; carbolic acid, also a strong poison which was implicated in deaths and serious injuries in a recent Sydney hospital mishap; aluminium which is linked with the development of Alzheimer's disease and allergies; and Thiomersal, a mercury-based preservative which is a known neurotoxin and whose inclusion in vaccination sparked a series of Congressional hearings which saw the US Government and the AAP (American Academy of Paediatrics) call for its immediate withdrawal from any vaccine product and which was withdrawn over two years ago in the USA from any over-the-counter medicines . It was also withdrawn from the American Hepatatis B vaccines, Engerix and HB Vax II, though their Australian counterparts which are still being injected into children here today, are only just being made mercury free or mercury reduced (though the old, mercury-laced stocks will be used up rather than being withdrawn from use).

## 3- Vaccines are contaminated with human and animal viruses and bacteria.

All childhood vaccines, apart from the Hepatitis B (which is genetically engineered and carries with it a different set of problems,) are cultured on either animal tissue, a broth of animal and/or human blood and blood products or the cell lines from aborted human foetuses. None of these culturing methods is able to guarantee an uncontaminated vaccine. In fact, it is well known that many foreign viruses and bacteria can and do contaminate vaccines. Almost none of these contaminants have been studied. The few which have been leave many parents concerned about the long-term effects of injecting these substances into their children. For instance, SV 40 (simian or monkey virus 40 – just one of 60 monkey viruses known to contaminate the polio vaccines) has been linked with cancers in humans; there is a chicken retrovirus which contaminates the measles and mumps vaccines called Reverse Transcriptase. This substance, an ancient non-human DNA code, is thought to switch on the HIV virus and cause it to become AIDS in humans; AIDS itself has been linked with a virus called SIV (Simian Immunodeficiency Virus) which contaminated both the polio and smallpox vaccines; the current MMR (measles mumps rubella) and other vaccines which contain bovine (cow) blood products are thought to be able to spread the human and always fatal form of mad cow disease, Creutzfeld-Jacobs disease, more readily than eating contaminated meat.

## 4 - Vaccines can cause serious immediate side effects.

As long as there have been vaccines, there have been reports of serious side effects following their administration. These side effects include (but are not limited to) convulsions and epilepsy, permanent brain damage, anaphylactic (life threatening allergic) reactions, Sudden Infant Death Syndrome (SIDS), retinal and brain haemorrhages (now being confused with Shaken Baby Syndrome) and death.

## 5 - Vaccines can cause serious long-term side effects.

According to medical reports, children are now less healthy than they have ever been before. More than 40% of all children now suffer from chronic conditions , something that was unheard of prior to mass vaccination. Vaccines have been associated with such conditions as Asthma, Eczema, Food Allergies, Chronic Ear Infections, Insulin Dependent Diabetes, Arthritis, Juvenile Rheumatoid Arthritis, Autism, Attention Deficit Disorder, Ulcerative Colitis, Irritable Bowel Syndrome, Hyperactivity, Schizophrenia, Multiple Sclerosis, Cancer and a raft of other chronic and auto-immune conditions which are experiencing dramatic rises in incidence.

## 6 - Vaccines do not necessarily protect against infectious diseases.

For many years, parents were told that once a child was fully vaccinated, they would be protected for life. That has now turned into a series of life-long boosters that are still not able to protect either children or adults from infectious diseases. For the very real risk of both short and long-term side effects from vaccines, parents are asked to allow their children to be given vaccines that at best, will provide a temporary sensitisation to illnesses and at worst, can make their children more susceptible to both opportunistic and infectious illness. As evidenced by the recent whooping cough outbreak in SA, the only Australian state which actually records vaccination status in cases of infectious illness, 87% of all those who contracted whooping cough and whose vaccination status was known were fully and appropriately vaccinated. In fact, Australian government statistics have shown that the majority of outbreaks in Australia occur in those who have been either fully vaccinated or were too young to be fully vaccinated.

## 7 - Doctors, as paid salesmen for vaccine products, are no longer considered to be trustworthy arbiters of their safety and effectiveness.

Doctors are currently receiving several payments from the government to push vaccines. These include $6 for reporting vaccinations to the Australian Childhood Immunization Register (ACIR), a national database which tracks vaccination status in our children and which has been called "a back-door Australia Card"; $18.50 on top of their Medicare rebate for vaccinating a child on time; and a bulk payment at the end of each year based upon them having a practice vaccination rate in excess of 80%. These payments can add up to many tens of thousands of dollars in a busy inner-city practice. As a result of this grossly unethical situation, doctors can no longer be thought of as objective when it comes to this issue. Parents no longer trust that their doctors will recommend that they vaccinate simply because it is the best thing for their child rather than the best thing for the doctor's bottom line.

## 8 - Pharmaceutical companies have paid for almost all vaccine research to date.

Just as the tobacco companies paid for corrupt and incorrect research which purported to show that tobacco and tobacco products were safe for human consumption, so too the pharmaceutical companies have paid for and produced almost all of the research into vaccines. While the Australian government continues to spend literally hundreds of millions of dollars a year in promoting and implementing vaccination campaigns (an example is the $292 million earmarked for vaccination against Meningococcal this year alone!) and little or no money on independent research, parents will continue to mistrust the research that has been performed by vested interests. After all, companies are by their very definition commercial concerns which are motivated by profit. There is nothing that would make a pharmaceutical company intrinsically more ethical and therefore more trustworthy than a tobacco company.

In addition, it is a little-known fact that the Therapeutic Goods Administration (TGA), the government body which licenses and registers vaccines and other medical products, does not perform any tests whatsoever to verify pharmaceutical company claims of safety or effectiveness.

## 9 - Doctors and health professionals rarely if ever report vaccine reactions.

In discussions with representatives of both ADRAC (The Adverse Drug Reactions Advisory Committee) and the SAEFVSS (Serious Adverse Events Following Vaccination Surveillance Scheme), the two government bodies charged with keeping track of reactions to vaccines and other drugs, the AVN's representatives were informed that less than 10% of all adverse reactions are ever reported. This means that the government's claims of vaccine safety are admittedly 90% incorrect. In addition, the AVN's adverse reactions database currently contains details on more than 800 serious adverse vaccine reactions. Not one of these reactions was ever reported by the doctors or health professionals involved. Parents cannot rely on data with that wide a margin of error when they are dealing with the health and well-being of their children.

**10 - Some childhood illnesses have beneficial aspects and therefore, prevention may not necessarily be in the best interests of the child.**

Measles, for example, has been used in Scandinavian countries to successfully treat such autoimmune conditions as eczema and many studies have performed which show that children who do not contract measles naturally as a child are more likely to suffer from certain cancers later in life. In addition, recent studies have shown that contracting the common childhood illnesses help to prime and strengthen the immune system in a way that vaccinations just cannot do. This priming means that children are much less likely to suffer from the now common allergic and autoimmune conditions that plague them today. Conditions such as asthma, diabetes and cancer. In addition, vaccinated mothers cannot confer passive immunity to their children even if they have contracted the wild form of the disease. This immunity used to protect all children during their vulnerable first months and years. Now, a vaccinated mother will give birth to a child who will be susceptible to these infections when, prior to vaccines, they would normally have been immune.

Vaccination is a medical procedure. It should never, ever be mandated. Nor should there ever be any coercion, financial or social penalties for those parents who have chosen, as is their right under the law, not to take the above risks on behalf of their children.

Unvaccinated children continue to be among the healthiest children in our society. They are no more the carriers of disease than any other healthy person. It is the government's responsibility to do the necessary research to ensure that procedures they are recommending for all Australian families are as safe and effective as they possibly can be. It is also their responsibility to keep vested interests honest. On both counts, this government has failed in its duty of care to our most vulnerable resource – our children.

Any one of the many points raised above deserves critical examination and public discussion and the parents who ask these questions deserve respect, not vilification."

Reprinted with kind permission of Meryl Dorey, President of the Australian Vaccination Network, Editor of the Informed Voice Magazine - Your Health, Your Rights, Your Options. For more information contact www.avn.org.au.

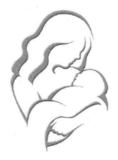

# Chapter 13 - Breastfeeding Tips

Begin to breastfeed your baby immediately after birth. The reflex to suck is the strongest during the first hour after birth. Let your birthing team know of your intention to breastfeed immediately after birth.

## How to Breastfeed Your Baby

1. Select a peaceful setting.
2. Find a comfortable position using good arm and back support.
3. Do not hurry. Remember you have all the time in the world.
4. Pick up your baby before your baby gets fretful.
5. Drop your shoulders, breath out and relax as you put your baby to your breast.
6. Make sure that your baby is latched onto your areola, not just your nipple. Your baby's nose and chin should be touching your breast. This is the correct latch.
7. Remain quiet, speaking to your baby after the feeding.
8. Do not interrupt your feeding time with your baby.
9. Enjoy the time you have together. Make it peaceful and relaxing for you both.
10. Drain your first breast completely before starting on the next. Smaller babies may want to take a short rest in between breasts. In the first month feed your baby whenever your baby cries for as long as your baby needs to feed. This will adjust your supply to your baby's exact needs. Put your watch and schedules away and relax.
    - Breastfeeding is an acquired skill for both baby and mom, just like playing the piano or driving a car. Make sure you have professional breastfeeding support for the first day and first week. If you are in a hospital, ask for the lactation consultant to see you immediately. Nurses

are too busy to take this special time for every mother and often do not have professional training in breastfeeding.

- It can take four to six weeks to get mom and baby used to breastfeeding. Your body is going through a tremendous adjustment and so is your baby. Make a commitment to stick to it. Don't give up if you become faced with a problem. There are times during this period when it will seem impossible, but once it all comes together breastfeeding will become second nature to you both. As you both become more skilled each feeding will take a shorter duration, you will be producing a greater volume of milk and your baby will need fewer feedings.
- Be persistent and patient.
- If you have not yet attended a breastfeeding clinic or meeting, find a Lactation Consultant and arrange for her to come out to talk to you. She will quickly assist you in answering any questions and taking care of any problems you may have while they are small.
- Help your partner to become comfortable with your breastfeeding by answering any questions he may have and letting him know how much easier, healthier, and inexpensive breastfeeding will be for your family. Talk about what he can do to nurture and love your baby so that he feels included. Let him know that you plan to express your milk and create a milk bank so that he can experience feeding baby as well.
- Do not let anyone in the hospital or at home feed your baby water. Water will reduce your baby's desire to suck as your baby's stomach will feel full. Make sure everyone who comes in contact with your baby realizes you are breastfeeding and that no one is to feed your baby but you.
- Feed your baby as often as possible in the first few hours after birth. Most babies will then sleep for a solid twenty-four hour period in the first day and night and you will want to give your baby the assurance and warmth of your breasts and heartbeat and to insure that your baby gets as much colostrum as possible. Practice makes perfect in every case of breastfeeding for both mother and baby.
- Your baby's stomach is the size of your baby's closed hand at birth and for the first month your baby will need to breastfeed frequently.
- Breastfeeding is extremely soothing to your baby. Toddlers say breastmilk tastes better than ice cream, one more fact owing to its great popularity with babies.
- If you and your baby are having any difficulties in the hospital use one of their electric breast pumps and have your baby cup fed, syringe fed,

or finger tube fed with your breastmilk until you work these problems out. This is especially important for premature babies. Premature babies have their own unique breastfeeding challenges and a quick conversation with a breastfeeding consultant will speed both of you on your way. Breastfeeding and Kangaroo Care for your premature infant can help to avoid many of the difficulties a premature baby has with adjusting to its new world.

- Let everyone know you plan to work through any difficulties.
- Keep pacifiers, soothers and bottles away from your breastfed baby.
- Leave your top and bra off as much as possible for the first two weeks to facilitate ease of breastfeeding, to air dry nipples and to increase bonding with your baby.
- Always express a few drops of breast milk and let the drops dry naturally on your nipple after each feeding. The milk will sterilize and heal any lacerations on your nipples.
- If you find your baby is choking due to the volume of milk and the speed of your letdown reflex make sure your baby is breastfeeding in a sitting up position. If you lean back in your chair you will slow the flow of your milk.
- After each feeding, make sure to remove any excess air by burping your baby. One way is to hold your baby upright on your lap while putting one hand under your baby's neck and head. Use your other hand to press or pat firmly on your baby's back. You can also put your baby over your shoulder or lean your baby across your knees.

## Correct Latch

Almost all breastfeeding difficulties are caused by your baby not being correctly latched onto your breast.

1. Use your nipple to tickle the chin.
2. Wait for a wide open mouth with the head back and bring your baby's entire body toward your breast and body.
3. Latch on with your baby taking your entire nipple and most or all of your areola surrounding your nipple. Your nipple should be far back into your baby's mouth. Your baby's nose and chin should be touching your breast.
4. If you wish to hold your breast while latching on make sure your hand is well back from the nipple.
5. To detach place your finger in your baby's mouth to reduce pressure as the baby is removed from your breast to help prevent scraping of your nipple.

## Positioning

Sit your baby up to breastfeed as soon as possible to reduce the stress on your arms and shoulders. Your baby will also enjoy sitting to breastfeed as this will reduce choking and makes swallowing much easier. You can feel how difficult it is to swallow when you are lying flat on your back and how much easier it is to swallow when you are in an upright or semi-upright position.

Experiment with new positions as much as possible. Be creative. Be comfortable. If your breasts are smaller consider investing in a breastfeeding pillow. This is a curved pillow that fits around your waist and helps to hold your baby closer to your nipple; the breastfeeding pillow will ease shoulder and neck pain as well.

Different positions include the cradle hold as described above, the football hold is good for c-section recovery as you hold your baby beside you with her legs up and there is no pressure on your surgery site. If you wish to feed your baby lying down make sure your baby's head is raised higher than the body using a small pillow or your arm to raise your baby's head up.

You can even breastfeed your baby upside down, with your baby's feet towards your head as you are lying down. This is a good position to use if you have a blockage in your breast duct.

## Engorgement

Engorgement can happen three to five days after your baby is born or later. This can be the most painful part of breastfeeding and luckily engorgement lasts for only a few days. This is a great time to express and save your extra milk by collecting and freezing. When your milk comes in your breasts will feel hot, you may have a fever and you will probably feel miserable. You can achieve quick relief with a bag of frozen peas placed upon your breast. Take Tylenol to reduce pain and fever.

- Have a hot shower and let the water run over your breasts. Apply hot packs to your breasts. Once the hot packs have been applied you can more easily express your excess milk. Only express enough to release the pressure or you will be creating even more milk. Don't worry, engorgement only last a few days and your body will quickly respond to the feeding needs of your baby.
- Cabbage leaves molded into your nursing bra and then frozen can be worn for a short time between feedings for comfort during engorgement.
- When feeding your baby make sure your baby always completely empties the first breast before you go on to the next one. This way you can

eliminate any blockages in your breast before they build up. Completely draining the first breast will also increase your milk supply and will increase the weight of your baby at a faster rate.

- Use cold packs on your breasts sparingly as they will reduce your milk supply. You are better off to apply heat and express any extra milk to obtain relief. Pump off only to the point of comfort or else you will increase your milk supply and you will find your breasts filling up again within a half hour.

- If you find any hard lumps the size of a pea in your breast at any time after you have completed a feeding, press down hard on the lump with your thumb or finger and gently work the lump towards your nipple. Make sure your baby sucks that breast completely dry at the next feeding.

- You may find yourself waking up in the middle of the night completely soaked. Keep a supply of clean towels folded by your bed and use one underneath you as you sleep. It is much easier to wash a towel than to change and wash the sheets. Soon your milk will be established and the leaking will stop.

## Expressing Your Breast Milk

The best time to express your milk is in the middle of the night or first thing in the morning, before the first feeding. Creating a milk bank can give you peace of mind and the knowledge that you will always have an abundance of milk on hand for your baby. When expressing your milk only one-third of the available milk supply is expressed, only your baby is able to remove the remainder of your milk. When you express your milk that you are naturally increasing the supply available to your baby as supply increases naturally upon demand throughout your breastfeeding relationship.

Begin by gently massaging your breast for one minute. Visualize your baby feeding to trigger your mind to bring down your milk. Cup your breast with your fingers on the bottom and your thumb on the top of your breast close to the edge of your areola, which is the brown colored part of your breast. Always keep your thumb in the same position and gently press down and out toward the nipple. Once you find the best spot to release your milk keep your thumb in exactly that spot every time you express your milk. Use the same milking rhythm your baby uses by pressing down and out in short intervals.

You can use a Playtex with plastic liner for breast milk freezing and temporary storage in your refrigerator. When expressing your milk you can use any clean container you happen to have by you.

The first time you express your milk you may express only one ounce or drops. Continue to add to this amount throughout the day and freeze what you have collected at the end each day. Do not add warm milk to frozen milk. Each time you express your milk it will become easier and faster and as you progress in your breastfeeding you will collect more milk each time. To defrost frozen breastmilk place the plastic bag into a glass of warm or hot water. It should unthaw within a few minutes. A microwave should never be used to defrost breastmilk.

Handle your breasts gently at all times especially when you are fully engorged. Your breasts bruise easily. It is not force that brings your milk down but a gentle milking action that will allow you to gently remove milk.

## Nipple Care

- Always express the last few drops of milk and allow them to air dry naturally on your nipples. Your milk contains natural healing substances that will condition your nipple.
- Never allow your baby to suck on your nipple. For a correct latch your baby must have your nipple and your areola all the way into its mouth.
- Breastfeeding should never hurt. If you are feeling any pain, talk to a female breastfeeding specialist right away.
- Never allow your breasts to become chapped by rubbing against wet fabric or breast pads. Keep an extra pair of cotton breast pads in your purse so that you can quickly change them should they become wet. Washable, cotton breast pads allow air to more easily circulate around your nipples.
- Your nipples will lose much of their sensitivity after the first month and this sensitivity will come back once you have finished breastfeeding.
- Remain braless as much as possible when at home to keep your nipples dry and to help with the circulation in your breasts.
- Apply a warm compress for five minutes after a feeding then keep nipples continually dry between feedings.
- Vitamin E oil can also be applied to heal cracked nipples.
- Never use hand or body lotion as they contain ingredients that can harm your baby or give them distaste and put them off feedings.
- Breastfeed on the side with the least pain to start as your baby will suck more vigorously on that side first. As your baby sucks your nipple will feel better once the milk begins to flow. Your breast milk contains natural healing substances that will work to heal your nipples as your baby feeds.
- If dry or chapped nipples are a continual problem go to a breastfeeding

clinic or neighborhood La Leche League meeting near you to make sure you are properly latching on your baby and that the positioning is correct for your baby.

# Thrush

In Smart Medicine for a Healthier Child: A Practical Reference to Natural and Conventional Treatment for Infants and Children, you will find a guide to conventional, homeopathic, herbal, nutritional, prevention and acupressure therapy for many disorders. Thrush shows up as white patches inside your baby's mouth, making it difficult for your baby to feed. General information about this condition includes information on related conditions like canker sores, warts, diaper rash, yeast infections and diabetes, which sometimes predisposes to thrush and yeast infections, and nutritional deficiencies that contribute to a general susceptibility to viral, bacterial, or fungal infections in general and of the skin specifically, as well as foods not to eat in case of a yeast infection.

Eating foods rich in vitamin A (carrots), B complex (whole grains, eggs, green beans), vitamin C (tomatoes, greens) folic acid (greens), and eating a whole grain, lean meat, legume, and non-sweet vegetable diet which is inhibitory to yeast can help as well. Refined sugar, flour, and cereal products as well as sweet vegetables and fats, foods which yeast thrives on, should be omitted. Diluted apple cider vinegar with water can also be included for both the baby and mother. Licorice root and ginger tea are also part of the recommended herbal treatment. Contact a breastfeeding consultant for treatment for you and your baby should thrush appear.

# Increasing Your Milk Supply

Every mother worries at some time if she has enough milk. Real signs of milk scarcity include a dry diaper two or three hours after feeding or not producing at least eight really wet diapers in a twenty-four hour period. Talk over your concerns with a breastfeeding professional if this should happen.

- Keep in mind that your baby may be crying for reasons other than food. Read the newborn section on crying in this guidebook to find out what your baby's unique sensitivities are and work to temporarily reduce either light, sound or movement in your baby's environment. And you can help your baby to practice self-calming techniques such as sucking on hands, fingers and wrist, focusing and favorite body positioning instead of continual feeding for calming. Training your baby to use other methods to self-calm rather than using your breast to calm will release both of you from becoming completely dependent on each other.

- The easiest way to increase your milk supply is to breastfeed more frequently.
- Give both breasts at each feeding. Make sure each breast is drained before starting on the next one. If your baby still seems hungry, put your baby back onto the first breast to help her get every last drop.
- Do not rigidly limit your baby's sucking time. The composition of milk changes as she sucks the thirst quenching foremilk, like skim milk, and then the more concentrated hind milk, which is like cream. This hind milk is very satisfying for your baby and can only be accessed by her when the breast is completely drained to the end.
- Don't offer a bottle instead of the breast. Even if she sucked so recently that you are sure there cannot be any more milk for her there will always be a little left and preventing her from taking it will make your breasts fill up more slowly.
- Don't offer a bottle along with the breast. Frequent breastfeeding will sustain her and cue your breasts to make more milk.
- Breastfeed as often as your baby likes. It doesn't matter if she has to suck very often to keep satisfied, with each feeding your supply is automatically increased. And as your baby grows you will automatically begin to produce greater amounts of breast milk.
- Bringing your baby to bed with you during the night and breastfeeding two or three times during the night will increase your supply. The milk you produce during the night while resting is also very rich and satisfying for your baby.
- Take a walk out in the fresh air before breastfeeding to relax.
- Some mothers have had great success with drinking small amounts of stout beer to restimulate supply.
- If you must leave your baby, express before you leave and while you are away if necessary. The best bet is to find a way to bring your baby with you when you go. You will be surprised at how many people love to see a newborn and your baby will enjoy the outing as well. Breastfed newborns are easily comforted with a feeding and often sleep quite soon after content in your arms.
- Make sure you are eating properly, small meals of nutritional food, throughout the day.
- Keep your fluid intake up throughout the day and evening. The best way

to do this is to get a drink for yourself and sip on it every time you breastfeed.

- Rest is also important. Working a short nap into your day will give you the extra energy you need at this time.
- Herb teas that will help to increase your milk supply include blessed thistle, brewer's yeast, red raspberry leaf, marshmallow, or alfalfa for rich milk and added strength for mom.
- Make sure you are taking a mineral supplement. Your baby requires calcium most of all for the first few years. The calcium will continue to be drawn out of your body's stores and this can cause exhaustion in the mother. Taking good care of yourself during breastfeeding is well worth the end result of a happy mother and baby.

## Breastfeeding and Work

You do not have to quit breastfeeding because you are returning to work. It is possible to maintain your milk by breastfeeding your baby in the morning, late afternoon, the evening and night and on the weekends. Supplement with your personal milk bank for the day feedings or try to return home at lunch. Rent a portable breast pump and bring it to work. After you return to your career you will appreciate continuing breastfeeding for the rewards it gives to both of you.

Breastfeeding causes the hormone Prolactin to be released in your body, helping you and your baby to reconnect and attach at the end of the day. This hormone will also naturally relax and calm you. Your baby will receive these same benefits and more. Continuing your breastfeeding past your baby's first year will also boost your baby's immune system reducing or eliminating colds, flu and fevers.

## New Discoveries on Breastmilk

"Human breast milk has a full and balanced complement of minerals and vitamins, including calcium, phosphorus, zinc and vitamins B6, B12, C and D. Breast milk also contains a multitude of other components that help the baby grow and thrive. Some of them do double and triple duty. Here's a partial list:

**Secretory IgA** – This is human milk's most predominant antibody (Ig is short for immunoglobulin). At birth, babies cannot produce their own immunoglobulins. Instead they're protected by transplacental IgC that was transmitted in utero by Mom. But this lasts only a short time. Meanwhile, babies slowly develop the ability to make their own immunoglobulins. At 3 months, babies have a total antibody protection (transplacental IgC plus baby's own antibodies) that's only about 35 percent of what they had at birth. Breast milk's abundant supply of IgA helps fill the gap until babies can take over the entire job of protecting themselves. IgA acts like an intestinal "paint", coating the lining of the baby's gut and binding bacteria and viruses so they can't multiply. After a few hours, this IgA coating is sloughed off, digested as protein and excreted. Each time a baby nurses, he gets a new protective paint job. IgA is believed to play a key role in preventing diarrhea. In addition, whenever a mother is exposed to a bacteria or virus, her body manufactures a specific secretory IgA to protect her. If she's been exposed to a bug, in all likelihood so has her baby, but luckily, her environmentally specific IgA is secreted in her milk and transferred to the baby, bestowing a highly personalized protection.

**Lysozyme** – This enzyme acts like a powerful little Pac Man in the baby's digestive system. It chops up bacterial cell walls, powerfully and selectively gobbling up disease-carrying bacteria.

**Prolactin** – Until recently, scientists thought this hormone simply served to regulate Mom's milk production. Its presence in milk was considered a nonfunctional by-product. Research now supports the idea that prolactin helps activate and enhance the infant's immune system. A recent study published in Pediatrics hypothesized that the presence of prolactin and immunoregulatory substances in human milk (and their absence in formula) may be why breastfed babies have a lower risk of ear infection than formula-fed babies.

**Sialated Mucins** – These combinations of carbohydrate and protein with sialic acid help prevent viral diarrhea which causes more than 200 infant deaths annually in the United States. Recent research has shown that these mucins can pick up harmful viruses as they pass through the baby's intestine, then transport them out via the feces.

**Sialic Acid** (also known as n-acetylneuramic acid or NANA). – Besides enhancing the protective effect of mucins, NANA is important for normal cell membrane function and brain development. Breast milk contains about 5 to 10 times more sialic acid than formula does.

**Complex Oligosaccharides** – The blend of these carbohydrates in breast milk is unique. In addition to providing calories, these compounds prevent bacteria from binding to cell surfaces. Several studies have linked oligosaccharides to protection against urinary tract infections.

**Lactoferrin** – This protein delivers iron directly to where it's needed in the intestinal lining and sequesters unnecessary iron – an important function since many "bad" bacteria can't thrive without extra iron.

**Long-Chain Polyunsaturated Fatty Acids** – These fatty acids become part of the cell membranes of the infant's nervous system and are thus important to the continued development of the retina and brain. "Striking data indicates that these fatty acids are responsible for the enhanced visual acuity that has been shown to occur in preterm infants who received human milk compared to those who received formula," notes Judy Hopkinson, PhD., research assistant professor at the USDA Children's Nutrition Research Center at Baylor College of Medicine in Houston.

**Bifidobacterium** – These "healthy" bacteria, which are capable of destroying parasites, aren't actually present in mother's milk. Instead, certain carbohydrates present only in human milk encourage these bacteria to flourish in the baby's intestinal tract. The benefits of bifidobacterium were highlighted in a recent study conducted at the Johns Hopkins University School of Medicine: When hospitalized babies were given formula with added bifidobacterium, they have a substantially reduced incidence of acute diarrhea disease.

**Epidermal Growth Factor** – This hormone – like substance is important to the growth and maturation of the linings of the baby's liver, heart, intestines, kidney, pancreas and stomach."

Reprinted with kind permission from Fit Pregnancy Magazine, "Mother's Milk: What's in it for Baby?" written by Janis Graham author of Breastfeeding Secrets & Solutions.

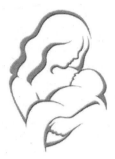

# Chapter 14 Newborn Care Tips

## The First Day

- Keeping your newborn close to you at all times during the first few weeks helps to build a bond of love and trust between you.
- Your baby is experiencing a profound adjustment as she is seeing, feeling and hearing our world for the first time. The best thing you can do for your baby is spend the day together in bed, only an arm's length away. Your baby has gone through a physically tiring labor and delivery. Your body also has gone through a tremendous strain, even more so if you have had any medical interventions with either your labor or delivery and your body is now providing colostrum and creating your breastmilk. Taking the next one or two weeks to rest will help your body to completely heal and for your milk supply to be created. Some cases of postnatal depression are rooted in the first few weeks home due to inadequate rest of the mother. Ask now and take all the assistance that is offered. You deserve to be cared for during this time.
- Not all women experience "love at first sight" especially if they have had a difficult delivery. This is completely normal. Don't feel guilty. Over time you fall madly in love with your precious baby.
- Your newborn is genetically designed to look more like your partner in the first few months of life. Most mothers are surprised at the great likeness in their babies to their partners and have trouble finding any likeness at all to their-self. Your baby will change to look more like you after the first month or two. This process is nature's way to assist both partners in continuing to bond to the new member of the family.
- Keep the lights in your home dim for the first day and noise to a minimum. Entertain any guests in your bedroom and ask all guests to keep their voices low. Don't feel you have to let anyone other than your

partner handle or hold your baby. Explain that just for today, you are keeping the house as quiet as possible.

- Breastfeed as often as you have the opportunity in your baby's first hours. Your baby will be awake for three hours or more directly after birth and will be the most alert for the longest time in the days to come. Some newborns will sleep for up to twelve hours after their first alert period.

- If you have any breastfeeding difficulties on the first day immediately contact your nurse, midwife, lactation consultant or breastfeeding mom to voice your concerns. Many breastfeeding challenges can be solved on the telephone. The most challenging problems are an improper latch or the position of the baby at the breast. Taking care of small problems before they become big problems will help you to easily become a great breastfeeding team.

- No matter how many pacifiers or soothers you are given for gifts do not use them. Studies are showing a direct link to pacifiers and ear infections in infants. A pacifier will cause your baby to be unable to communicate her needs to you and your baby will not be able to access it for herself when she needs soothing. Babies have also been shown to self-wean early when they are given pacifiers. If you are tempted to use one to forestall crying, see the crying and colic section of this guide for alternate methods for soothing a crying baby. Pacifiers also cause more difficulty with efficient feeding as your baby's jaw can become quite sore from the continual, instinctual sucking action caused by pacifiers. Babies who are given free and easy access to their hands in the first year rarely suck on their fingers or thumbs past the first year.

- Keep your baby's hands free from clothing and blankets at all times. Roll up the sleeves on jumpers and place the blanket only up to your baby's waist, leaving hands and arms completely free and available to your baby. If you are swaddling your baby keep those hands and arms free, wrapping the blanket under your baby's arms. From the first day, encourage your baby to suck on her fist, arm or fingers, just as your baby did in your womb. Fists, fingers and thumbs are available, clean and your baby will always be able to find them for comfort and security.

- Try a nail file for your baby's fingernails instead of clippers. Clippers are difficult to manage with a newborn and you run the risk of cutting the skin. You may need to file the nails on a daily basis as they will grow rapidly. Think of your baby's fingers and thumbs as your baby's best tools and keep them in good condition and available at all times.

- Give others the opportunity to hold your baby. Watch carefully how others hold, soothe and talk to your baby. You will get new ideas on how to be with your baby.
- Help your partner to change, hold and comfort your baby from the first day. Learn together what works best for your baby and share with each other your new discoveries of what works best.
- Set aside two days for friends and relatives to see your new baby. Having everyone over at once is easier for you and your baby.
- When placing your baby on the sofa, place your baby's back or side against the back of your sofa so that your baby feels more secure and less overwhelmed with such a large space around her. This also works well in the crib or cradle.
- Babies can be over stimulated by anxious parents trying to rock, burp, and soothe a newborn who just wants to be left alone. If your baby is fed, burped, dry, and warm, give your baby at least two minutes to vent and remove outside stimulus as in dimming the lighting, turning down the television or radio, and slowing down or stopping movement. You will find that your newborn craves a quiet environment when they are overtired or over stimulated. Peace and quiet is one of the greatest sources of comfort you can give your newborn in the first few months.

## Sleeping

Your baby has been used to living life as a night owl. Being rocked to sleep in the womb during the day as you carry on with your activities and becoming awake as soon as the motion stops and you lie down to rest at night. It will take up to two weeks for your baby to adjust to sleeping in the night and waking during the day. Be patient with your little one, in a short time this sleeping pattern will be adjusted.

Consider having your baby sleep beside you. Mothers have been sleeping in the same bed as their infants for centuries. Sharing your bed with your baby has many benefits:

- Your baby learns sleep and breathing patterns by being near you throughout the night. The carbon dioxide you breathe out also helps your baby to breath better and stimulates breathing as well.
- Breastfeeding in the middle of the night is much easier if your baby is in bed with you as it won't disrupt your sleeping patterns.
- It is less upsetting for your baby to sleep with you initially as your baby will not have to cry loud, or a long time to get your attention.

- Premature babies or other babies who were separated from their mothers at the hospital may attach more easily when they sleep with their mothers. This type of close contact will help your baby thrive.
- Safety first. Never sleep with your baby if you are drinking alcohol or taking drugs. Never let your baby sleep on a waterbed. Never place your baby on a bed that has a loose headboard or sideboards.
- If you feel uncomfortable, or if you, your baby or your partner are not sleeping well in this arrangement, set things up to suit yourself. You may want to use a cradle or bassinet next to your bed or to place the crib in your bedroom. A crib or cradle in your room beside the bed gives both of you the benefits from sleeping together for the first few months.
- Decide on your own time when to move your baby out of your bed. Have a small wicker basket or cradle at your bedside and gradually have your baby sleep there for part of the night. Make changes gradually so that everyone adjusts easily.
- Purchase a foam holder to assist your baby in sleeping on the side or back instead of on her stomach. You can also use a rolled towel or receiving blanket. This has been found to be the safest position for your baby while sleeping. Should your baby vomit or spit up while sleeping, there would be less risk of choking.
- Keep all toys, pillows, stuffed animals and the like out of your baby's crib or bassinet until your baby is at least one year of age to insure that fresh air easily circulates around your baby.
- With more babies sleeping on their backs now, you may want to place your baby on her tummy at playtime to help round out your baby's head.

## The Secret Language of Babies

For millions of sleep-deprived mothers and fathers around the world, this woman's findings could be a miracle. Priscilla Dunstan, a mom from Australia with a special gift, says she's unlocked the secret language of babies.

When Priscilla was a toddler, her parents discovered she had a photographic memory for sound. At age four, she could hear a Mozart concert on the piano and play it back note for note.

Priscilla says her gift has helped her hear a special "second language" beyond English, allowing her to detect moods and even diagnose illness. "Other people might hear a note, but I sort of get the whole symphony," Priscilla says. "So when someone's speaking, I get all this information that other people might not pick up."

That mysterious second language took on an astounding new meaning when Priscilla became a mother to her baby. "Because of my gift for sound, I was able to pick out certain patterns in his cries and then remember what those patterns were later on when he cried again," Priscilla says. "I realized that other babies were saying the same sounds."

After testing her baby language theory on more than one thousand infants around the world, Priscilla says there are five sounds that all babies newborn to three months say, regardless of race and culture:

1.  Neh, Neh, Neh  =  "I'm Hungry"
2.  Owh, Owh, Owh  =  "I'm Sleepy"
3.  Heh, Heh, Heh  =  "I'm Experiencing Discomfort"
4.  Eair, Eair,  =  "I Have Lower Gas"
5.  Eh, Eh, Eh  =  "I Need To Burp

These sounds are actually sound reflexes. "Babies all around the world have the same reflexes, and they therefore make the same sounds." If parents don't respond to those reflexes, Priscilla says the baby will eventually stop using them.

Pricilla recommends that parents listen for those sounds in a baby's pre-cry before they start crying hysterically. She says there is no one sound that's harder to hear than others because it varies by individual. She also says some babies use more sounds than others. The Dunstan Baby Language DVD is available for sale at www.dunstandbaby.com.

## Alternate Feeding

- Milk is ideal for calves but it is not a natural food for babies. Milk contains too little sugar and the wrong kind of fat. This protein makes indigestible solid curds in the baby's stomach. Babies under one year should not be fed on any kind of unmodified cow's milk. Babies need a breastmilk substitute for the entire first year if they are not breastfed.

- A new baby, especially one who is not breastfed, has few defenses against common germs. Formula, especially formula which is at room temperature is an ideal breeding ground for germs. So while she will pick up a few off her own fingers and deal with them perfectly well, she will pick up an overwhelming number from a bottle which has been left standing in a warm room. Gastroenteritis is still one of the most common reasons for babies being admitted to the hospital. Keep your baby's formula as free from bacteria as possible.

- To keep your formula free from bacteria, wash your hands before handling the formula or equipment. Use a sterile formula and keep the can tightly covered and refrigerated once it has been opened. Sterilize everything you use in measuring, mixing or storing the made-up formula. Sterilize bottles, nipples and nipple covers. Keep the formula cold until your baby wants it. Never put warm formula in a thermos or electric bottle warmer. Throw away any formula your baby leaves behind. Don't try to save that half bottle for next time and don't pour the now unsterile remains back into your jar of sterilized formula in the refrigerator, the remainder should be thrown out.

- If you do not have access to sterilizing equipment, cup feed or dropper feed your baby instead of using a bottle.

- When you combine formula powder or liquid concentrate with boiled water you are constructing food and most of your baby's drink. If you do it in exactly the proportions the manufacturer suggests, your baby will get the right amount of food and the right amount of water. Always follow the manufacturer's instructions exactly.

- You cannot make it better by putting in just a little extra powder or more thirst quenching by adding extra water. If you add too much powder, the formula will be too strong. Your baby will get too much protein, too much fat, too much salt, and not enough water. She will get fat because you are giving her too many calories and thirsty because you are giving her too much salt. Because she is thirsty, she will cry, and because she cries you will give her another bottle. If that bottle is too strong, she will be thirstier. The result can be a baby who cries a lot, does not seem terribly well or happy, puts on a lot of weight, and seems to need a lot of feeding.

- Never carry warm formula. It is a dangerously ideal breeding ground for bacteria. Carry the baby's formula icy cold from the refrigerator. Keep it that way by putting the sterile sealed bottles in an insulated bag or by burying them in ice cubes in a plastic bag. Warm the bottles as you need them by standing them in hot water from a thermos for a few minutes. If you are going to need more bottles than you can safely keep cold, measure formula powder into empty sterile bottles and seal. Mix with boiled water from a thermos as you need each one. Always carry at least one more feeding than you think you will need during the trip.

- How often do you feed a bottle-fed baby? Formula should be offered whenever the baby seems to be hungry and the feeding should only be stopped when eager sucking ceases. Don't try to push her to take more than she really wants. Your newborn's stomach is the size of her closed hand and will require small meals quite frequently for the first few months. Each baby has their own individual feeding requirements.

- A newborn is used to having her food needs continually replenished by transfusion feeding in the womb. While your baby gets used to this new method of feeding she may be hungry at irregular and frequent intervals. If you offer her a bottle whenever she seems hungry, she will only take the amount she needs. If she drinks it all you can assume she needed it. If she takes a little, the comfort of sucking and of your care will make her feel better. If she drinks none, what have you lost? If you meet these irregular demands willingly, they will stop by themselves in a few weeks. Do not put a newborn on any feeding schedule for this reason. After a few months your baby's unique feeding pattern will evolve on its own. So don't fall into the trap of thinking that if you feed your baby whenever she seems hungry she will get into the habit of demanding food frequently.

- Being physically close to you during feedings is just as important to the bottle-fed baby as to the breastfed baby. Always give her the bottle while she is cradled in your arms. Eating is a social occasion for us all including your baby. Choose a chair that supports your back and arms while your feet are flat on the floor. Always bottle-feed your baby with her head higher than her body in an upright or semi-upright position. Do not let your baby bottle-feed lying down as the fluids can accumulate in the ear canal causing ear infections. If you are bottle-feeding in your bed, place your arm under your baby's head to raise it up.

- When your baby stops sucking or when the feeding is finished you may want to burp your baby. Hold her upright against your shoulder, rub her back or pat it gently. If she has not burped after three minutes, she does not need to.

- If you find your baby either gaining too much weight or not gaining enough weight on your dairy-based formula you may want to switch to a soy-based baby formula for a thirty-day period. Many babies are milk intolerant and have difficulties digesting and eliminating the protein from a dairy-based formula.

## Diapering

- Make a game out of changing your baby's diaper and clothes. Smile at your baby. Laugh when your baby makes a big poop. Make this a fun time for your baby by taking an extra few minutes to talk to your baby, ask your baby questions and listen for responses, give a short massage on legs or arms, or to comment on your plans for the day. Your baby will cherish these times together with you and will also enjoy your undivided attention.

- Place an oversized mirror on the wall beside your baby's change table. Your baby will enjoy the reflection of both of you from the first day and will be fascinated at the changing images.
- Changing your baby in the bathroom will give you a mirror and water facilities.
- Use the corners of the last diaper to clean off. Use as many diaper wipes as necessary to be sure diaper area is completely clean, as anything left on the skin will cause a rash.
- If you are not using diaper wipes, a quick rinse in the sink can clean your baby's bottom in a minute.
- Don't change your baby when your baby is hungry.
- Expect your baby's first bowel movements to be black and tar-like, the next movements will be green, and then onto a seedy, mustard yellow. You may wish to use disposable diapers for the first two weeks of large bowel movements. Try buying the next size larger than newborn for complete coverage of these messy bowel movements.
- When possible, let your baby's bottom air dry by leaving the diaper and other clothes off for a short time by placing your baby on a disposable waterproof pad.
- If your diapers leak, change your diapers to a bigger size or to another brand.
- Breastfed babies sometimes go for a few days between bowel movements. As long as the bowel movement is still mustard yellow and has a soft texture, everything is fine.
- If your baby's skin is very sensitive try using natural aloe vera gel instead of powders or sticky creams. Make sure the gel is completely dry before putting diaper on to be assured that the protection will stay on the skin and not rub off on the diaper. You can also use this gel for prickly heat rashes.
- If your diaper cream is not working as you would like, switch brands until you find one you like. When you find one that works, purchase the largest size to save money. It is not necessary to use diaper cream all the time.
- Try natural corn starch, found in the grocery store, for a natural baby powder that helps prevent diaper rashes. Keep all powders away from

your baby's reach so that they are not accidentally breathed into your baby's lungs.

- Your baby should not continually have rashes. Check your diaper wipes or diapers to see if they are causing any sensitivity to your baby's skin. Look at the foods your baby is consuming: sometimes a rash is brought on by food reactions to dairy, fruits, bananas, etc. Remove or replace that food with another and see if the condition clears up. Disposable diapers can also cause sensitivity. If you are using cloth diapers try using a detergent purchased at a health food grocery store that has no dyes, phosphates, or chemicals. Make sure you presoak your diapers in dissolved Borax to change the acidic environment to alkaline.
- If a rash just won't go away, take your baby in to see your doctor.

## Help for Crying Babies

The world is a noisy, bright, and busy place for a newborn. If your baby cries excessively within the first 48 hours of life, please bring your baby to the doctor to make sure everything is ok.

For other crying: Feed your baby, change your baby, make sure your baby is nice and warm, especially head and toes. Then you can:

1. Turn down the lights, turn down the sound and slow down movement and activity.
2. Hold me in my favorite position to help me to look out and focus on a light or blank wall.
3. Roll up my sleeves and bring my hands close to my mouth so that I can look at or suck on my hands, fingers and thumbs.

These steps will help your baby to use their instinctual skills to calm down and stop crying. Practice these self-calming skills daily with your baby and within a short time your baby will automatically use these natural skills to calm and relax.

## Crying & Colic – How to Help Your Baby to Stop Crying

All crying in the first year should be attended to immediately. Crying is your baby's only method of communication with you. If your newborn is crying constantly throughout the day and night, take your baby to the hospital or to your doctor immediately for a thorough checkup to assure yourself that your baby is well.

Some newborns are more sensitive to their environment than others. Should this be the case for your baby, the following suggestions may be of great assistance in creating a calm and soothing environment for you and your baby.

Thousands of parents have used the following self-calming method for their newborns with great success. Many see results in as early as seven days on the program. Expect your best results to come after you have used the program for thirty days. Never shake a crying baby as this can permanently damage the brain of your baby and will not stop the crying anyway.

"If your newborn has a pattern of crying non-stop for three or four hours, usually in the evening, wearing the both of you down, you may want to try the following to help your baby to stop crying. A newborn's world is loud, bright and similar to a nonstop ride at the carnival. Amazing new discoveries in the field of newborn care are now showing us that most crying in newborns is due to over-stimulation.

1. If, after your baby is fed, changed and warm, your baby is still crying, try taking your baby immediately into a quiet, dimly lit room. Turn down the lights, turn down the noise, and slow down your movement and activity.
2. Hold your baby's face and body away from you, facing your baby outward so that your baby can visually focus on something in the room.
3. Free your baby's hands and wrists from clothing and bring both of your baby's hands gently up towards your baby's face so that your baby can either focus on or suck on fingers, thumbs or wrist.
4. During this process it is best for the adult to remain silent.
5. As your baby begins to calm look for reasons for the crying. For example when has your newborn had the last opportunity to rest undisturbed or what activities came before the crying.
6. While you are in the quiet, darkened room either hold your baby or place your baby in her favorite body position on your bed with a hand gently massaging either their back or bottom of the feet. Look for signs of your baby beginning to calm on her own. Always make sure that your baby has easy access to her hands and wrists by rolling up the sleeves to the elbow and swaddling under the arms leaving the hands free.

As you get to know your baby, look to see what disturbs your baby the most when your baby is over stimulated. Is the most disturbing factor too much sound, too much light or too much movement?

If sound upsets your baby, stop talking, and turn down the volume on your television or stereo. Some babies find movement disruptive when they are over stimulated. If movement affects your baby, lay your baby down beside you and cease movement and activity until your baby begins to calm. If light disturbs your baby the most, immediately dim the lights or go into a darkened room. Using all three of these techniques at once in the beginning will allow you to obtain quick results while you are discovering your baby's unique sensitivities and abilities.

All newborns have instinctual self-calming techniques that help them to deal with the overload of new experiences they have every day. Given the opportunity your baby may instinctively begin to self-calm by doing one or all of the following:

1. Suck on wrist, hand, finger or thumb.
2. Focus visually on a blank space, white wall, or hand and fingers.
3. Have a favorite calming body position like laying on the back, or stomach, side or in a sitting up position.

- When you see that your baby is beginning to self-calm by either sucking, focusing or laying in a particular position, watch your baby without disturbing the process. If your newborn has had an extremely stressful day filled with activities, noise and movement you may see your baby work at self-calming for thirty minutes or more. By standing back and not giving your baby further stimulation at this time you are allowing your baby to create the confidence that comes naturally with a self-calmed baby. It is a great feeling for the parent to know that they are assisting their baby in what is natural for every baby.

- Make sure your baby has at least two quiet periods during the day to nap without noise or distractions. Highly sensitive babies need this quiet time everyday to de-stress.

- The best time to practice self-calming techniques with your baby is in the mornings. Late in the day and early evenings can be trying until your baby learns to rely on these skills. It may take four weeks or so for you and your baby to master these techniques and your patience and guidance will greatly assist your baby in developing this skill at this time. During the first thirty days you will have some setbacks and there may be times when your baby is unable to self-soothe. This is natural and should be expected as both parents and baby develop this skill.

- Using pacifiers, automatic swings, car rides, rocking and walking or whatever else you may have heard of will only delay your baby's ability to develop this skill of self-calming. It is far preferable to take the time now to assist your sensitive baby to be calm and relaxed. Many parents wish they had these skills for themselves. In our fast paced world we all need to acquire the ability to relax and release the stress from our busy days.

- Often your baby will cry today because of the activities that happened the day before. Review where you went and what you did the day before and then reduce your daily activity level with your baby for a week or two while you are helping your baby with self-calming. Have the groceries sent in, delay errands or have someone else pick things up for you, pay your bills by mail and postpone whatever isn't essential during this period of time. This will help you to see what unique combination of sensitivities your baby has and will give you more immediate results with the program.

- As a protective skill your baby is also born with an instinctual ability to play "possum". Many people are amazed to see a baby peacefully sleeping in the midst of a noisy party, such as a christening or baby shower. In this instance your newborn is using an innate ability to shut out all distractions in an attempt to deal with an overload of stimulus. Using this skill is very tiring for a baby as it takes much more energy than sleeping. You will probably notice that your sensitive baby will be more agitated the next day as a result of the party. Babies will usually lose the skill to play "possum" from the age of six weeks to three months. This skill can be lost in a day when a previously happy and content baby becomes a crying baby. This is the end of the honeymoon period for most babies and parents and an excellent time to encourage your baby to self-calm using this natural, instinctual ability.

- Some mothers stop breastfeeding at six weeks if they have been using extra feedings to calm their newborn. Breastfeeding is a natural way for your baby to use instinctual self-calming methods as it combines sucking, focusing and favorite body position. Unfortunately soon the mother begins to resent continuous and prolonged feedings and the infant soon resents being offered food as the only solution for every problem, just as we would if someone put food into our mouth every time we were frustrated, angry or tired.

- Researchers once felt that at this critical period of time, when your baby is no longer able to play "possum", the baby was going through a growth spurt. After measuring hundreds of babies during this period, and no measurable growth appearing in the babies, we have discovered that the reality is that your baby is actually losing one skill, the ability to play possum and tune everything out, to rely more frequently upon and to develop the other instinctual skills of sucking, focusing and body positioning for self-calming.

- As you get to know your baby's unique sensitivities you may notice that if your baby is overly sensitive to loud noises or talking when overtired, your baby will also probably love music in any form when rested and relaxed. Then communicating with your baby through nursery rhymes and songs, lullabies, sharing your favorite music or buying a musical mobile for your crib, children's tape player and tapes or any musical toy will help you to experience your baby's world from their point of view.

- You can get to know the baby who is sensitive visually by noticing the shadows on the wall as your baby is watching the various light patterns, talking about the light that has caught your baby's eye, pointing out the stars at night or a street light in the evening. Your visually oriented baby may enjoy going to movies, watching you while feeding, sitting up on your lap and being able to see what is going on in the world around them. By catching your baby's attention when your baby is noticing something you will have a short opportunity to explain what it is or what it does. Taking 30 seconds at a time to notice what your baby sees and talking about it will encourage your baby's curiosity and your baby will feel more connected to you.

- A baby who is sensitive to activity may prefer being placed in a favorite sleeping position with a firm hand placed on the back or stomach for a few minutes before sleep. This may calm your baby and will slow down the activity level. Your baby will greatly enjoy being free of encumbrances and holding devices. The best place for this baby is a large blanket on the floor with plenty of encouragement to move about. This baby loves to have you on the floor beside them when playing and will enjoy any kind of physical activity when rested and calm.

- Your baby may have one or any combination of the above sensitivities. You can easily discover for yourself the unique way your baby perceives our world by becoming aware of these traits in your baby. Teach your family and alternate caregivers these self-calming methods and let them know what you've discovered about your baby and they will be as amazed as you will be with the effectiveness of this program.

- As you get to know your baby, you will begin to know how long your baby can cry before your baby is unable to calm. When settling your baby down for a nap your baby will initially protest by crying. Each day you bring your baby in for a nap the time of crying should become shorter. If you feel your baby may be crying for a particular reason or wish to ease your mind, go in and pick up your baby while staying in the room. If your baby immediately stops crying you will know that your baby was able to self-calm and that you may have entered the room too soon. If your baby takes a long time to calm after you have picked your baby up then your baby has a shorter time in which they can cry before they will self-calm. It is a great advantage to a baby to be able to put themselves to sleep without crutches like pacifiers, bottles and frequent visits throughout the evening, and your baby's skill at falling asleep alone will increase with self-calming practice.

• As your baby increases her skill level of self-calming and you learn what your baby's sensitivities are, you will find that it becomes easier to know what your baby needs from you at any particular time. When your baby has been fed within the last two hours, is dry and clean and warm, you will look at your watch to see when the last time your baby had a chance to "de-stress" from daily events by napping. We often forget how noisy, bright, and fast-moving our world is. Everything is new to your baby and giving your baby a chance to slowly adjust to the world can be the best gift you give your newborn.

• A crying baby adds stress to your family relationship. Take the time to carefully watch your baby for signs of self-calming and encourage your baby in each step. Working together as a team will create a calm and loving environment for you both and your baby will learn self-calming techniques that can last a lifetime."

Reprinted with kind permission from Dr. William A.H. Sammons. For further study of this amazing new research on why babies cry you can read The Self-Calmed Baby, by William A.H. Sammons. Every baby should come with crying instructions. This program often yields more than a 90% success rate when field tested with new parents and new babies.

## Shaken Baby Syndrome

"The combination of a crying baby and a frustrated parent or caregiver can be deadly.

## Why do babies cry?

Crying is the only way babies have to tell us that they need something. They might need to eat, to have their diaper changed or to be held. The baby could be too hot or too cold or in pain. Sometimes babies cry because they need to release some tension of their own. Crying is normal. The amount of time a baby spends crying varies with age, health and temperament.

## Why do parents and caregivers become frustrated and angry?

Crying is an annoying sound. It is supposed to be. If it was a pleasant sound, crying would be easy to ignore and the baby's needs would never be met. Unfortunately, parents and caregivers are not always able to stop the crying. When a baby cries a lot and is not easily consoled, the parent or caregiver may start to doubt their own abilities to care for the baby. Lack of sleep and other life stresses can increase the feelings of helplessness and frustration. Sometimes parents or caregivers believe that a crying baby is misbehaving on purpose.

## What can a parent or caregiver do?

Stay calm. A frustrated or angry parent or caregiver will have a hard time getting a baby to settle down. If feeding, changing, walking, rocking and cuddling have not worked, the baby should be gently placed in a safe place and allowed to "cry it out" for a few minutes. The parent or caregiver can use the time to relax and calm down before making another attempt to console the baby.

# NEVER SHAKE A BABY!

Shaking a baby in a moment of frustration can cause serious harm or death. When an infant is shaken, the head jerks back and forth rapidly causing the brain to slam repeatedly against the inside of the skull. Blood vessels in and around the brain are damaged and begin to bleed into the brain and into the space between the brain and the skull. The bleeding and swelling of the brain causes pressure to build up inside the child's head. The resulting damage can cause permanent disability or even death. Because babies have weak neck muscles and heavy heads, even a few seconds of forceful shaking can cause serious damage to babies and small children. Children under one year of age, especially baby boys, are most at risk. Older children can also be hurt if they are shaken hard.

## What happens to shaken babies?

As many as one third of the victims of Shaken Baby Syndrome die. The survivors often suffer lifelong disabilities due to the brain injury such as:
- blindness.
- paralysis.
- mental disabilities.
- growth and development problems.
- seizure disorders.

Some babies who are shaken also have broken ribs or arms from being held tightly by the person doing the shaking.

## How much shaking is dangerous?

Victims of Shaken Baby Syndrome have been violently shaken. Their injuries are at least as severe as that which would occur if an infant was dropped from a high building. Although it is unlikely that severe injuries would occur from tossing an infant in the air playfully or bouncing a small child on a knee, parents and caregivers should always consider the fragility of an infant's brain and the need to support the head and neck. Even minor injuries to a baby's brain can have life long consequences.

It is never okay to shake a baby!

## How can Shaken Baby Syndrome be prevented?

Providing information on the care and normal development of infants is an essential element in the prevention of Shaken Baby Syndrome. It is also important that parents and caregivers understand that the feelings of frustration they experience are common and very normal. Learning how to handle those feelings can be made easier through community education and support programs.

It is important that all caregivers know that SHAKING IS DANGEROUS. Parents should ensure that babysitters and daycare providers are informed and experienced."

Reprinted with kind permission from the Saskatchewan Institute on Prevention of Handicaps. Copyright 2006

# Baby's First Bath

- You can wait to bath your baby until after the umbilical cord has fallen off.

- Wash your baby's hands and face each morning with a warm washcloth and keep your baby's bottom clean with your spray bottle of water or a quick rinse in the sink, keeping this area spotlessly clean especially after a bowel movement.
- When you feel ready you may wish to bring your baby into the big bathtub with you for the first bathing experience. Lean back against the tub with your thighs at a slant. Place your baby on the slant of your legs with only your baby's feet in the water. Talk and smile at your baby to reduce any tension from this new experience. Use a washcloth to bring water up from the tub and over your baby. If you like, breastfeed your baby while in the tub to make this a memorable experience for both of you.
- Later, when bathing your baby, you may wish to wash your baby's hair over the sink or small tub while she is still clothed, and then continue to undress and bathe the rest of your baby. This can reduce the fear of this new experience and will keep your baby warmer and more comfortable.
- Europeans bathe their babies two or three times a week instead of daily to prevent dry skin. You baby will not require a daily bath until she starts crawling.

## How to Install Your Car Seat

Most parents believe they are doing all they can to prevent their children from being injured in a car accident. Transport Canada found in their own study that six out of ten children are at risk because of neglect to use or incorrect use of car seats and seat belts. Police, the province and public safety groups have launched a zero tolerance blitz to make certain children are safe. Drivers who fail to make sure the children in their car are secured safely risk incurring tickets for violation of safety laws and they must attend mandatory re-education instruction sessions.

The most common problem with poor car seat safety is caused by improperly installed tether anchor bolts. A tether bolt is required in all Canadian provinces and is a bolt attached to the rear deck frame, not just the upholstery, of the car. A strap from the car seat is then attached to the bolt. Since 1989 all cars in Canada must have a hole drilled by the manufacturer that accommodates this bolt. To find the bolt, look for the plastic dome that covers it. To install the bolt, just pop out the dome. If you have an earlier model than 1989, then you would have to take your vehicle in to a service center to have the hole drilled.

Deciding which seat to purchase is largely a matter of determining your child's weight: Infant Car Seats are for babies weighing less than 9 kg/20 lbs and should be rear facing with the infant's head protected and supported by the back of their infant seat. It is a Canadian law that your child be securely fastened into their car seat in the correct manner. NEVER PLACE A CAR SEAT OR A CHILD IN THE FRONT SEAT OF A VEHICLE THAT IS EQUIPPED WITH AIRBAGS.

Convertible Forward Facing Seats are for children between 9-18 kg/20-40 lbs. The seat must be properly anchored to the car with a tether strap and bolt plus the car seat belt. The harness straps go over the shoulders and not under the arms. The shoulder straps are secured with a shoulder harness clip supplied by the manufacturer and placed at chest level. Again, this is law that your child is secured in this manner.

Sales personnel are trained to offer you the best product available but the most important person for knowledge is yourself. Don't assume you know how a car seat works or any other product that involves a child's safety. Always read your car owner's manual for complete and proper instructions.

# Establishing A Night-Time Ritual

- Remember even a newborn, one day old, can sleep for six straight hours.
- When your baby awakens during the middle of the night, do not change the diaper unless you absolutely have to.
- Keep all lights dim. Use a night light close to your bed, in the hall and in your baby's room for easier night-time navigation.
- Do not talk to your baby in the middle of the night and your baby will soon realize that night is for sleeping not visiting.
- Tell your baby that it is time to sleep when you lay your baby down.
- If your breasts become completely engorged at night, and your baby has not yet awakened, wake your baby up gently and feed. You are a breastfeeding team and you deserve to be comfortable as well. Or keep a clean glass by your bedside and express just until you feel comfortable.
- Expect at least one middle-of-the-night feeding for the first few months. Keeping your baby in your bedroom will help everyone get back to sleep faster.
- Many babies will cry out in the middle of the night and then settle themselves down. Wait for two minutes before you attend to your baby to see if your baby goes back to sleep on their own.
- Have your baby in your bed or beside your bed for ease of feeding at night.

To avoid turning on the lights, place a finger on your nipple and bring baby's mouth to your breast, as this will help your baby to latch on in the dark.

- Do not keep your baby awake during the day, hoping this will tire your baby out at night. An over-tired baby has a hard time getting to sleep. Let your baby sleep throughout the day and early evening if needed. It is not necessary to awaken your newborn for feedings during daytime naps as this practice conditions your baby to relate sleeping and eating. Your newborn needs uninterrupted sleeping periods to recharge fully and will awaken naturally when ready.

- Sleep during the daytime, preferably at least two naps, a nap in the morning and in the afternoon of a few hours duration in a quiet room or in your arms, is the best answer for most newborns. Make your baby's nap the most important time of the day and work to schedule other events around this time. This way your newborn will receive the periods of quiet and calmness a very new baby needs, and you will get a much needed break to recharge your batteries as well.

- Sometimes babies awaken during the night because their feet are cold. Putting a pair of socks on under a sleeper or nightgown can help to keep your baby at the right temperature all night long.

- Establishing a night-time ritual can also consist of a warm bath, feeding or rocking, playing a wind-up mobile or music box, reading a story or anything you choose to do consistently before bed.

# Jaundice

For mild jaundice, breastfeed your baby as much as possible in the first three days to eliminate or prevent jaundice. The colostrum that is created before the breast milk is designed to help your baby to expel the first black, green and then yellow stools. Do not feed your baby water as a remedy for jaundice. Place your baby on the carpet in front of a sunny window with only a diaper on for ten or fifteen minutes a day, shading your baby's eyes from direct sunlight, or place your crib or cradle in a sunny spot in the room. Consult your health team if your baby has lethargy, is refusing to feed or any other symptoms associated with jaundice.

# Cradle Cap

- For flakes, massage a little mineral oil into hair and shampoo out. If your baby has a tougher case, where you can see patches of yellow or brown scales in the scalp, purchase a high quality Primrose Oil, from your health food store. Puncture the gel caps and massage into your baby's scalp every day for one week.

- Olive oil, castor oil, or calendula cream can also be used topically to remove the scales. Apply directly onto your baby's scalp, massage in and let soak for 15 minutes. Apply firm but gentle pressure with a fine toothed comb, loosen and comb out the scales and then shampoo.
- Some mothers are finding that reducing their own sugar intake when breastfeeding can help tremendously in reducing or eliminating cradle cap.
- Some doctors recommend a weak solution of cortisone cream for extreme cradle cap that spreads in small patches to the body. Cortisone will thin the skin if used extensively.
- Gently comb or brush your baby's hair every day even if your baby has only fine down. This will help with scalp circulation.

## Talking to Your Baby

Studies show that talking to your baby from the first day can help to create a more alert baby. Ask your baby questions and wait for a response. Say, "Did you have a good sleep?" Then wait 30 seconds for a response. Then come up with your own answer for your baby.

- Use your baby's proper name whenever possible in your sentences.
- Copy out loud the various grunts, squeaks and sounds of your baby. Your partner will be excellent at this. Soon you will have a language together all your very own. Whether you speak your baby's language of grunts and squeaks or your language of words, your baby will feel very much a part of your world. This is called mirroring and is a delightful game for newborns and babies.
- The following research on the development of your baby's brain details the tremendous advantages for our babies when we take the time to talk with them.

## New Discoveries on the Development of your Baby's Brain

"A baby's brain is a work in progress, trillions of neurons waiting to be wired into a mind. The experiences of childhood, pioneering research shows, helps form the brain's circuits for music, math, language and emotions.

You hold your newborn so his sky-blue eyes are just inches from the brightly patterned wallpaper. ZZZZt a neuron from his retina makes an electrical connection with one in his brain's visual cortex. You gently touch his palm with a clothespin; he grasps it, drops it, and you return it to him with soft words and a smile. Crackle; neurons from his hand strengthen their connection to those in his sensory-motor cortex. He cries in the night: you feed him, holding his gaze because nature has seen to it that the distance from a parent's crooked elbow to his eyes exactly matches the distance at which a baby focuses. Zap; neurons in the brain's amygdala send pulses of electricity through the circuits that control emotion. You hold him on your lap and talk and neurons from his ears start hardwiring connections to the auditory cortex. And you thought you were just playing with your kid.

When a baby comes into the world her brain is a jumble of neurons, all waiting to be woven into the intricate tapestry of the mind. Some of the neurons have already been hard-wired, like the genes in the fertilized egg, into circuits that command breathing or control heartbeat, regulate body temperature or produce reflexes. But trillions upon trillions more are like the Pentium chips in a computer before the factory preloads the software. They are pure and of almost infinite potential, unprogrammed circuits that might one day compose rap songs and do calculus, erupt in fury and melt in ecstasy. If the neurons are used, they become integrated into the circuitry of the brain by connecting to other neurons: if they are not used, they may die. It is the experiences of childhood, determining which neurons are used, that wire the circuits of the brain as surely as a programmer at a keyboard reconfigures the circuits in a computer. It determines whether the child grows up to be intelligent or dull, fearful or self-assured, articulate or tongue-tied. Early experiences are so powerful, says pediatric neurobiologist Harry Chugani of Wayne State University that "they can completely change the way a person turns out".

Once wired, there are limits to the brain's ability to create itself. Called "critical periods" they are windows of opportunity that nature flings open, starting before birth, and then slams shut, one by one, with every additional candle on the child's birthday cake. . . Neurobiologists are still at the dawn of understanding exactly which kinds of experiences, or sensory input, wire the brain in which ways. They know a great deal about the circuit for vision. It has a neuron-growth spurt at the age of 2 to 4 months, which corresponds to when babies start to really notice the world, and peaks at 8 months, when each neuron is connected to an astonishing 15,000 neurons. A baby whose eyes are clouded by cataracts from birth will, despite cataract-removal surgery at the age of 2, be forever blind. . . The implications of this new understanding are at once promising and disturbing. They suggest that, with the right input at the right time, almost anything is possible. But they imply, too, that if you miss the window you're playing with a handicap.

The language brain has a learning window from birth to ten years. Circuits in the auditory cortex, representing the sounds that form words, are wired by the age of 1. The more words a child hears by 2, the larger her vocabulary will grow. Hearing problems can impair the ability to match sounds to letters.

What we can do about it: Talk to your child – a lot. If you want her to master a second language introduce it by the age of 10. Protect hearing by treating ear infections promptly. As the basic circuitry is established a baby is primed to turn sounds into words.

The more sounds a child hears, the faster she learns language, according to Janellen Huttenlocher of the University of Chicago. Infants whose mothers spoke to them a lot know 131 more words at 20 months than did babies of more taciturn, or less involved caregivers. At 24 months, the gap had widened to 295 words. It didn't matter which words the caregiver used, monosyllables seemed to work. The sound of words, it seems, builds up neural circuitry that can then absorb more words, much as creating a computer file allows the user to fill it with prose. There is a huge vocabulary to be acquired, says Huttenlocher, and it can only be acquired through repeated exposure to words.

The logical brain has a learning window from birth to 4 years. Circuits for math reside in the brain's cortex, near those for music. Toddlers taught simple concepts, like one and many do better in math. Music lessons may help develop spatial skills.

What we can do about it: Play counting games with a toddler. Have him set the table to learn one to one relations, one plate, and one fork per person. Giving preschoolers piano or singing lessons has been shown to increase the children's ability to work mazes, draw geometric figures and copy patterns of two-color blocks. It is suspected that when children exercise cortical neurons by listening to classical music they are also strengthening circuits used for mathematics. Music, says a team of researchers from UC Irvine excites the inherent brain patterns and enhances their use in complex reasoning tasks. Early musical training develops spatial intelligence, the ability to visualize the world accurately and this skill later translates into complex math and engineering skills. "Early music training can also enhance a child's ability to reason." says Irvine physicist Gordon Shaw.

The greatest effect a parent can have on emotions comes through "attunement" or playing back a child's inner feelings. If a baby's squeal of delight at a puppy is met with a smile and hug, if her excitement at seeing a plane overhead is mirrored, circuits for these emotions are reinforced. Apparently, the brain uses the same pathways to generate an emotion as to respond to one. So if an emotion is reciprocated, the electrical and chemical signals that produced it are reinforced. But if emotions are repeatedly met with indifference or a clashing response – those circuits become confused and fail to strengthen. The key here is repeatedly, one dismissive harrumph will not scar a child for life. It is the pattern that counts, and it can be very powerful. In one of Stern's studies, a baby whose mother never matched her level of excitement became extremely passive unable to feel excitement or joy."

Reprinted with kind permission from Newsweek, February 1996, Newsweek, Inc. "Your Child's Brain: How Kids are Wired for Music, Math and Emotions", Sharon Begley.

## The Emotional Development of Your Baby

Your baby's primary emotional development is set quite firmly into place during the first three years, as shown in the studies of Burton White at his Harvard University Project and by other top researchers today. Emotions such as love, joy, excitement, compassion, empathy, bonding and attachment are laid down like tiles upon the floor forming a foundation for your baby's emotional life.

You can help your baby to recognize and acknowledge feelings by mirroring back to them as they occur. Your baby's excitement can become your excitement. Your baby learns empathy when you soothe their cries. Your baby understands compassion when you respond to feeding, changing, and comfort needs. Your baby experiences love as you gaze deeply into each others eyes. Anger and fear seem to need no introduction to your baby and both seem to be permanently installed from day one as a part of the fight or flight instinct.

The best ways to enrich your baby's emotional development are as follows:
1. Hug your baby often.
2. Crawl Baby Crawl – Find ways to let your baby explore the world safely.
3. Always respond to your baby's coos and cries.
4. Sing to your baby.

5. Create discipline by making meals and naps predictable.

A recent television special entitled, This Is Your Child, gives a common sense approach to your baby's emotional and intellectual development. For information on this program call 1-888-447-3400. This program can also be accessed on the internet at www.iamyourchild.org.

## Playing With Your Baby

Speak to your baby. Tell your baby how big she is growing. Explain what you are doing, where you are going, noises your baby hears, names of things, how things work, as well as names of the people around you. Every time you communicate with your baby, your baby learns a new word or sound of your language. Just as when you are learning a foreign language, you learn much about what someone is communicating with you by words, gestures and tone of voice.

- Play the alphabet game with your baby by sounding out the letters of the alphabet. Start with the sound of A and finish with the sound of zzzzzz. Your baby will love to hear certain letter sounds like sssss, and will be fascinated to hear the sounds of your language one at a time. Babies love to hear this game over and over and it may win you your first smile.

- When you feel excited, whether about a certain outing you will be taking or an event that is happening show your baby your excitement. Your baby will feel your excitement and will then feel included in what is going on around her.

- When you see that your baby is entranced with something visually, notice it yourself and talk about the item. By observing the behavior of your baby you will begin to build a bridge of communication between the both of you.

- Babies love to dance with you, cheek to cheek, to your favorite music.

- Give your baby a gentle massage over her clothes upon awakening from a nap.

- Smile at your baby whenever you remember and you will have a baby who smiles at you.

- Kiss your baby as often as you like. All babies thrive on love, affection and praise, and most especially when this encouragement comes from you.

- Sit your baby up as much as possible when your baby is alert, this gives your baby a much better view of the world. Make sure you are supporting your newborn's head and neck.

- When your baby is stretching after a nap, gently tug on her arms and legs along with her.

- Bundle up your baby in a blanket and go for a walk around the block. Some babies are calmer and sleep better after some fresh air.
- Play music for your baby whenever possible as music increases the development of your baby's brain. A portable Fisher Price tape recorder is an excellent way to have music in the bath, the kitchen and all around the house and outside. Experiment with different types of music and you will probably find that your baby has quite a sophisticated taste in music and will especially like any music that you enjoy.
- Cuddle up together with your baby on your chest. Have a short nap or just daydream together.
- Play with your baby's arms, legs, toes and fingers.
- Your baby loves to look at bright lights. Go out in the evening after dark for a short walk and look at the stars and street lights.
- Turn the radio up in the car and sing to your baby.
- Make silly faces or silly noises.
- Play pat-a-cake or little piggies with your baby.
- Bring your baby around to different rooms and explain what you are doing. Babies love to play in a basket of freshly dried clothes and they can help to make that endless chore go more quickly for you.
- The first year with your baby is full of excitement, exploration and exhaustion. Spend as much time as you can down on the floor with your baby and encourage your partner to do so as well. Your baby will show you things you never thought possible. Talk to her, hold her and love her. By the end of that first year, she is ready to pull away and be more independent and it gets progressively harder to cuddle her and just hold her. Once she learns to walk, she wants to move. Enjoy those first few months of closeness because it will never be just that way again.

## Play with a Purpose

Reprinted with kind permission from Gymboree Parent Play Guide the world's leading play program combining fun, learning, activity and music in an interactive environment for parents and babies. Expect to have just as much fun, or more, as your baby. Developmentally appropriate classes are offered for newborns through five years of age. Gymboree has experience with over 1,000,000 families worldwide in over 375 locations around the world.

When your child approaches a new physical activity, praise and support him no matter what his level of mastery. Encourage him to try activities again, be close to offer help and support, and applaud his accomplishments enthusiastically. Remember there is no right or wrong way for a child to approach a new physical activity, as long as it is safe! Keep in mind that all activities in this guide are to be done under parental supervision.

When helping children to walk, support them around the torso or hold the back of their clothing. Doing so frees their arms for better balance. This applies to children from early walkers taking their first steps to older children trying a balance beam for the first time.

Make car trips more fun by having several familiar musical tapes handy. Younger children will be soothed by the familiar music; older ones will join in and sing for entertainment.

Enhance every activity you participate in with your child by promoting language development. Talking while dressing and bathing helps even young babies understand the rhythm, flow, use and meanings in language. With older children, name and count objects and colors, identify directions like going up or down and spatial concepts like through, on, over, as you and your child experience these activities.

Maintain eye contact with your child when he is trying a new activity, such as crawling through a tunnel. For instance, place yourself at one end of the tunnel and look through to the child to provide a familiar landmark and friendly encouragement.

For a baby who is about to crawl, place hands under the soles of baby's feet and gently support them while crawling. Let baby push against your hands, rather than you pushing baby. This works especially well when baby is attempting to crawl up a small incline.

Let your children crawl and walk barefooted as much as possible. Doing so strengthens foot muscles and provides tactile stimulation.

Simplify for success. Make sure you are providing play opportunities in which your child can be successful. As she develops self-confidence and mastery of an activity, begin to build in new and more advanced challenges.

Remember, each child develops at his own pace. Encourage your child's curiosity and willingness to test new feats. This will promote self-esteem and build confidence, the most important accomplishment of all!

Practice makes permanent. Remember that children learn through repetition. Activities that they enjoy may be repeated again and again, each time with a little more mastery than the last.

Young children learn by integrating information gathered through their sensory systems. The following play ideas will assist your baby in learning the developmental tasks of balance, motor planning, spatial awareness, and will help to develop your baby's auditory, visual and tactile systems. A play program at Gymboree will show you how to make the most of play with your baby. Most programs feature over forty pieces of gym equipment created especially for babies and crawlers to help you to play safely as well. Here are some parent interactive activities you can use at home:

Place sofa cushion and pillows on the floor. Lay baby on tummy with arms and head over the edge of cushion. Baby can push up with arms in preparation for crawling. Scatter cushion as an obstacle course for baby to crawl over and around.

Using the leaf from your dining room table, you can set up a slide for your baby. Place the leaf on the edge of couch or chair for a gentle incline. Make sure it is on carpeting or padding for safety. Supervising carefully, place baby on tummy to slide feet first. Baby can also crawl up the leaf as a ramp.

Fill your big tub with water for baby to sit in and play with a variety of toys. Use various sponges and cloths to wash your baby for different tactile experiences. On a summer morning, place a small tub outside and fill with water. By afternoon, the water will be warm enough for play. Never leave your baby unattended in close proximity to water.

Make baby's first tunnel out of a large box. Lay the box on its side and cut off ends Be sure to remove all staples. Maintain eye contact with baby as you place him inside the tunnel.

Place baby on tummy on top of a ball and gently roll ball in all directions. Older babies may sit upright atop ball. Baby Soccer: Hold child by the trunk and gently swing him to kick ball with his feet. Ball may be kicked to another person or against a wall.

Blow bubbles for babies to watch and to reach. As baby sits up, hold bubble on the end of a wand for him to reach out and pop. Bubbles are a great activity to encourage eye tracking and eye-hand coordination.

Place baby on back on center of small sturdy blanket. With two adults each holding two blanket corners, gently and careful swing baby side to side and head to foot. Lift the blanket up and down for even more fun.

To enhance self awareness, place shatterproof mirrors at floor level so baby can see himself. Play peek a boo by covering the mirror with a scarf.

Stand an inner tube on its side and place baby inside with upper torso resting on tube in crawling position. Baby will push up in preparation for crawling. Place toys and balls within easy reach for baby to play with.

Hide a music box or alarm clock under a blanket. Let baby react to the noise and look for the source of the sound.

Let baby focus on a beam of light and track it on the wall. For more challenge move the light in circles and at a different pace, fast and slow.

Play peek a boo by putting a scarf or cloth over your head. Eventually your baby will experience cause and effect by pulling the scarf off himself.

## The Magic of 21

Researchers have long known the magic of 21 in learning a new habit or in releasing an old one. New research is now showing this number is valuable for babies and children as well. If we carefully watch our children at play we notice that they will repeat the exact same activity for an exact number of times. This number is 21 times.

This number correlates directly to the exact number of times an activity needs to be repeated in order to be permanently placed into the neural pathways of the brain. The first pathway is like a line, then a tiny path, then a road, then a two-lane highway, four-lane highway, and finally an expressway into the mind. When the expressway or neural pathway is completed, after 21 times, a myelin coating then covers that pathway making it permanent. The myelin coating speeds conduction of thought whenever that task needs to be repeated. Thus as your baby begins to laboriously open and close that tightly clenched fist it becomes easier and easier with each attempt.

If the baby or child is interrupted before a set pattern of repetitions have occurred in a new learning experience, the pathway will not be completely developed, frustrating the child. To allow the greatest amount of learning to take place it is often best to allow them to decide the exact amount of attempts needed to complete a task. So when you watch your baby in a new play activity, watch for the magic of 21 and you will see the pride and satisfaction in your baby when the task at hand has been successfully completed.

## Eye Contact

It takes a few months before your baby will establish direct eye contact with you when you speak. Watch for moving arms and legs to assure you that indeed your baby is listening to you.

Your newborn has perfect vision of twelve to eighteen inches at birth. Just far enough away to see your smiling face as you are feeding or holding your baby. Make sure you have everyone keep their faces back at least 12 inches to avoid overwhelming your baby in the first few months.

Your baby will focus mainly on your hairline and will be memorizing the contrast of your skin and hair. Your baby is using many of her senses to get to know you and your partner besides her vision with her sense of touch, sense of smell, sense of taste, and hearing. Your baby can hear you even though she is not looking directly at you. Don't let it discourage you from talking to your baby as much as you can.

# Baby Sign Language

"Baby Sign Language are simple physical gestures which your hearing baby can use to communicate with you until they have conquered the intricacies of spoken language.

Babies naturally resort to using their body language, facial expressions, noises, cries and gestures in order to communicate with you. Baby Sign Language is just an extension on what your baby can already do. Look at how easily babies learn to wave 'goodbye' and how much they love action songs. By introducing a few simple signs your baby will be able to tell you what she is thinking about-More food; I want milk; look at the dog, etc.

By having this wonderful resource at your fingertips you and your baby are able to have meaningful conversations you would have missed out on if you had waited until she was able to talk.

Studies have shown that babies aged between six and thirty months benefit the most from using Baby Sign Language. Children learning English as a second language and speech delayed children have also benefited. In summary, Baby Sign Language fills the communication gap until your baby has mastered spoken language.

## Benefits for Baby

One of the key aims of Baby Talk is to help babies to talk earlier. There are a number of associated benefits from using Baby Sign Language, all of which relate to the fact that your baby has a two way communication channel available to them much earlier than would otherwise be possible.

**Greater Independence**: The fact that your baby can tell you about what they want, when they want it, gives them a greater sense of confidence. This is because they have a greater understanding of their environment, and because they have another means of learning, associating and understanding, hence they feel freer to explore. You are providing a 'scaffolding" for your baby's learning experiences, whereby your baby makes new discoveries knowing you are there for support and encouragement.

**Given more attention**: The methods used to teach signs are all based around focusing your attention on your baby and being more observant. You will begin to think in more detail about your daily routines with your baby, and identify opportunities for learning.

**Helps babies to talk earlier**: The studies on Baby Sign Language indicate that signing babies end up well ahead of their non signing counterparts in terms of language development. The physical movement involved with signing helps to concrete objects, emotions and concepts into an infant's mind, and makes it easier for them to associate the spoken word. Your baby is able to see and feel the word, as well as hearing it.

**It's Fun**: Your baby becomes very enthusiastic about learning new signs as it means they can connect with you more often about many different things. They are able to take charge of their own education by indicating to you what they want to know more about. These interactions work very well as they are initialed by your baby. Learning animal signs is always lots of fun because it's an opportunity to be really animated and make lots of noise. Singing songs and nursery rhymes is also an excellent way of teaching signs. Build lots of animal signs into your daily routines.

## Benefits for the Parent

There are significant benefits for you as a parent or caregiver, and probably the main one is the amount of fun you and your baby will have throughout. Speak to any parent who signs with their baby and you will quickly come to understand that even small steps forward in communicating can make a significant difference to your relationship with your infant.

It's hard to describe the amount of fun you will have communicating with sign language. From the moment you see your baby repeat their first sign, you will be hooked.

The best part is that there are hundreds of opportunities every day to teach signs. Even a simple trip to the supermarket becomes an opportunity to teach signs for dog and cat in the pet food aisle. A trip to the zoo allows you to reinforce your animal signs, and have lots of fun making all the noises and gestures along side the real thing. A visit to a farm or pet show can be even better, as it allows you to get up close to the animals.

**Additional benefits include**: Baby Signs help you with bonding with your baby, you can share the wonder of your baby's new world and you will find it reduces frustration. Just the fact that your baby can tell you more about what they are thinking, means that they are less likely to be frustrated in their attempts to communicate with you. Overall, what you get out of Baby Sign Language is determined by the effort you put in to learning with your baby. Make the learning experience as fun as possible by making use of everyday objects and environments."

Reprinted with kind permission from Babytalk Ltd. For more information contact: www.baby-talk.co.nz .

## More Baby Signs:

The First Sign for All Babies: Waving Bye-Bye.

Nodding head up and down for yes.

Shaking head for no.

Saying "Shhh" with your fingers across lips for sleeping.

Showing empty hands to say all gone.

Bird – Flap one or both arms.

Flower – Sniffing gesture.

Fish – Open and close lips making smacking noises.

More – Tap the index finger of one hand into opposite palm.

Duck – Keep fingers straight and open and close like a beak.

Cat – Stroke the back of your arm with fingers like stroking a cat.

Dog – Open your mouth and pant.

Bottle/Drink – Put thumb to your lips and tilt your head as if drinking.

Eat – Two fingers pressed against lips.

## Startle Reflex

When moved abruptly from place to place, your newborn may startle. Pick up your baby slowly and gently, and have others do the same, holding your baby close to your body when you are moving.

When putting your baby down for a nap or onto the change table, keep your hand on your baby for a minute after. If your baby startles, gently press both of baby's arms together with your hands, hold for 30 seconds and gently reassure your baby.

## Sneezing

Your baby sneezes to remove the amniotic fluid from her lungs and to blow her nose. This can happen off and on for a few months. Your baby may also have a raspy sound to the breathing from the amniotic fluid as well.

# Ear Infections

Research is now showing that liquid can travel into the middle ear while feeding causing ear infections. Liquid is more likely to drain out and away from the ear canal when the baby is fed in a semi-upright position. If you are lying down during breastfeeding simply place your arm under your baby's head to raise the head sufficiently. Keep your baby's head raised above the body for all feedings, especially during the last few moments to avoid this problem. A bottle to bed can also contribute to ear infections and should be avoided.

Multiple ear infections, continual colds and a runny nose could be a sign of a dairy intolerance. Changing to a soy baby formula for a short time will give you an excellent indication if this is the case.

Ear infections that are not treated can cause serious hearing loss for your baby. A middle ear infection can make a baby or child extremely ill very quickly, with high fever and great pain. A doctor should be called immediately if an ear infection is suspected. Treatment, usually with antibiotics will prevent a burst ear drum and possible damage to hearing. The child may be ill without making it obvious that his ear is the cause; this is why a doctor will always examine an ill child's ears even if they do not appear to hurt.

# Dehydration

Dehydration in a newborn is cause for alarm. After the first week you will want to see at least six very wet diapers per day. Dehydration usually occurs as a result of vomiting and loose bowels. Signs of dehydration include listlessness, lack of tears, flaccid muscle tone, or being unable to rouse your baby. Always keep an eye on how many wet diapers your baby has during the day as this will let you know how much fluid your baby is ingesting. An extremely dehydrated newborn will show a marked depression on the top portion of her head. If you see any of these danger signs, immediately call your doctor or nearest emergency department.

Dehydration is not the simple drying out that the name suggests. A body that is seriously short of water cannot maintain the complex and delicate balance of chemicals on which it's functioning depends. This is why a baby or very young child who has become dehydrated will not instantly be restored by a drink of water. He will need a careful mixture of chemicals and fluid dripped directly into his bloodstream. Diarrhea and/or vomiting, especially if accompanied by fever, makes a baby very liable to dehydration because each episode may deprive his body of more fluid than his last drink put in. The younger the child; the greater this risk. Babies under six months with symptoms of dehydration should be seen by a doctor as a matter of medical urgency.

# Eczema

Infantile eczema tends to run in families. There will probably be a close relative susceptible either to eczema or to some other allergic complaint such as hay fever or asthma. Like all allergic conditions it will be made temporarily worse by anything which upsets the child. The vast majority of children outgrow the eczema by the age of three.

The disorder usually begins with bright red scaly and itching patches on the cheeks. There may well be scurf on the scalp and this may lead to bad patches of itchy rash behind the ears. Occasionally the rash spreads to cover large areas of the body, but it is usually concentrated in the moist creases; in the groin, behind the knees, etc. When the eczema is very active, acute inflammation makes the scaly red patches moist. Eczema itches continually and scratching will make the patches sore and may infect them. Your baby is likely to be desperately miserable.

Eczema is a signal that your baby may have intolerance to dairy as well as intolerance to certain perfumes and dyes in soaps and laundry detergents. Rather than first using topical treatment for this irritating skin rash look to see what in your baby environment may be causing this.

The first place to look is at your laundry detergent. Health food stores now stock laundry detergents completely free of phosphates, dyes, chemicals, perfumes and other additives. Take all of your baby's sheets, blankets, clothing, socks, and diapers and wash everything again in the new chemical-free detergent. Just by changing your laundry detergent you can often change the symptoms in a few days. You may also want to try a double rinse on your laundry.

Keep bathing to a minimum and bathe your baby in clear water only, using perfume-free soap or shampoo only in the last moments. If you have hard water in your city a Ecosave magnetic wash ball gives you rainwater softness in the bathwater by simply dropping the magnetic ball into the bathtub. This ball can be reused forever and has a lifetime guarantee.

You may also want to remove environmental irritants like tobacco smoke or pets from the home.

Buy cotton instead of polyester clothing for your baby.

Flax Oil massaged into the skin is very good for eczema and often helps clear the area immediately.

You can take all dairy products out of your baby's menu and substitute with soy infant formula to see if this is causing a reaction. If you are breastfeeding remove all dairy products from your diet while you are testing for intolerances. You should be able to track down the offending substance within a short while if the case is food intolerance.

Calendula cream used directly on the rash can be purchased in health food stores will help relieve your baby's discomfort. Eczema often shows up in children before asthma. Removing food and chemical intolerances from your baby's environment can help to forestall or eliminate asthma. See a homeopath for inexpensive creams and lotions to soothe and protect affected areas. Do not use any cortisone based skin creams on your newborn as it will cause permanent thinning of the skin in that area.

## Allergies and Food Intolerances

Sometimes a child who is allergic to a certain protein in her food or drink may produce symptoms that seems entirely unrelated to the digestive tract; eczema, for example or asthma or urticaria. Where food or drink leads to symptoms which are clearly digestive, it is often difficult to tell whether the problem is a true allergy or whether it is one of many kinds of intolerance. Many babies are having reactions to cow milk products. If you are finding any reaction to dairy based products switch immediately to a soy infant formula.

If breastfeeding you may want to eliminate dairy products from your diet and take calcium supplements. You may need to try a number of different soy products until you find the one that suits your baby best. Never use regular soy milk products or rice milk as a infant formula for the first year as they will not provide adequate nutritional support. You must use a formula specifically designed for an infant for your baby's first year.

Allergic reactions and intolerances to a food product can show up in a variety of ways such as projectile vomiting, continual diaper rash, wheezing, continual runny nose, drowsiness, swollen eyes, darkened circles under the eyes, lethargy or non-stop crying, or any out of the ordinary symptoms that may occur after your baby has eaten.

Rice milk is a great-tasting, easy to digest and nutritional substitute for cow's milk after the first year when your baby is having three solid meals a day. You can ask any grocery or health food store to stock it for you.

# Solid Food

Everyone has different advice about when to feed baby solids. Most doctors now recommend that your baby should be mainly on breastmilk for the first year. Many mothers begin to supplement with solid foods after the first six months.

- Your baby may go from breastfeeding to rice cereal, to canned baby food to table food. Or your baby may go from breastfeeding straight to drinking from a cup and eating food from the table.

- All food prepared for your baby should have a wet texture as your baby does not have sufficient saliva to swallow dry food.

- Bland, digestible pure rice cereal mixed with breast milk or applesauce and water is a good first food.

- Vegetables and fruits should come next. Start with vegetables first since babies who become accustomed to the sweetness of fruit sometimes turn up their noses at veggies. Sweet potatoes and yams make an excellent first vegetable. Peel and boil and then mash with a fork adding some of the boiled vegetable water. Carrots and peas are also a good first food and can be easily prepared in the same manner.

- Homemade soups are also a great first food. Slightly overcook the soup to make a soft consistency. Adding rice or noodles to the soup gives variety. If you don't have time to start a soup from scratch, start with a can of soup or a bullion cube and water and add fresh vegetables to it as you go along.

- Introduce one new item at a time, a tablespoon each day. Don't be surprised if your baby spits out the first taste. If your baby rejects a new food, wait a few days and then try again. Your baby is learning new textures as well as new tastes.

- Try not to imitate your baby's faces when you are offering new foods. Often your baby is reacting to the new texture of the food rather than the taste of it.

- Get creative, mashed potatoes, mashed bananas, instant oatmeal, Cheerios, animal cookies and Ritz bits when the teeth come in. Then later, canned or homemade soups, frozen peas, fruits, etc. Watch your baby for clues. Your baby will let you know when she is ready for different tastes and textures. Have your baby join the family at the table when you are eating. Her natural curiosity will serve her and you well.

- If you are breastfeeding you may want to make the decision to continue breastfeeding beyond the first year of your baby's life.

# You and Your Baby – The First Six Months

"One day you will find that you have stopped regarding your baby as a totally unpredictable and therefore rather alarming novelty and have begun instead to think of him as a person with tastes, preferences and characteristics of his own. When that happens you will know that he has moved on from being a "newborn" and has gotten himself settled into life. Nobody can date that moment except you. An easy birth, close satisfactory contact immediately after it, and a good fit between his needs and your expectations will all tend to bring it forward. Postnatal depression, feeding difficulties, or a baby who needs handling in a way that does not come naturally to you will all tend to keep it back. But whether he is settled at two weeks or at two months, that moment will come.

A settled baby is a manageable proposition. You can tell how they like to be handled even if it is not the way you would choose to handle them. You know what to expect from even if it is the worst. You know what frightens your baby even if it is almost everything. Once your baby is settled you know what you are up against. Instead of trying to survive from hour to hour, get through another day, avoid thinking about another week, you can begin to work and plan for reasonable compromises between your baby's needs and those of everyone else.

Your baby will make it increasingly clear that apart from food, the prime need is for people who are the constant caretakers. Your love for your baby may still be problematic, but the dawn of this attachment to you is a matter of sheer necessity. If your baby is to survive, he has to attach himself to you and ensure that you take care of him. As these first few weeks pass, his interest in people becomes increasingly obvious. Your face fascinates him. Every time it comes within his short focusing range he studies it intently, from hairline to mouth, finishing by gazing into your eyes. He listens intently to your voice, kicking a little when he hears it, or freezing into immobility as he tries to locate its source. Soon he will turn his eyes and his head to see who is talking. If you pick him up, he stops crying. If you will cuddle and walk him, he remains content. Whatever else he likes or needs, he clearly likes and needs you. You can begin to have some confidence in yourselves as the parents of this new human being.

But in case these settled responses to your devoted care are not enough to keep you caring, your baby has a trump card still to play: smiling. One day he is studying your face in his intent and serious way and he scans down to your mouth and back to your eyes as usual. But as he gazes, his face slowly begins to flower into the small miracle of a wide toothless grin that totally transforms it. For most parents, grandparents and care givers, that's it. Few adults can resist a baby's new smiling. Even the most reluctantly dutiful visitors have been known to sneak back to the crib side to try for one more smile all for themselves.

When the baby smiles it looks like love, but he cannot truly love anyone yet because he does not know one person from another. His early smiles are an insurance policy against neglect and for pleasant social attention. The more he smiles and gurgles and waves his fists at people, the more they will smile and talk to him. The more attention people pay him, the more he will respond, tying them ever closer with his throat-catching grins and his heart-renderingly quivery lower lip. His responses create a self-sustaining circle, his smiles leading to your smiles and yours to more from him.

There is no harm in assuming that these enchanting early smiles are meant for you personally. They soon will be. It is through pleasant social interaction with adults, who find him rewarding and therefore pay him attention, that the baby moves on from being interested in people in general to being able to recognize and attach himself to particular ones. By the time he is around three months old it will be clear that he knows you. He becomes both increasingly sociable and increasingly fussy about whom he will socialize with. He is ready to form a passionate and exclusive emotional tie with somebody and you are elected.

If a baby's mother is available at all most babies select her for this first love. But the blood-tie doesn't automatically qualify you for the privilege. It has to be earned, not just by being your baby's mother but by mothering him. And mothering does not just mean taking physical care of the baby. The love he is forming is not cupboard love rooted in the pleasures of feeding. Babies fall in love with people who mother them emotionally, talking to them, cuddling them, smiling and playing with them. If you had to share your baby's total care with one other person and you handed over all the physical tasks, using your limited time for loving and play, you would keep your prime role in your baby's life. But if you used your time to meet his physical needs, leaving the other person to be his companion and playmate, it would probably be that companionable adult to whom he became most closely attached. Of course your baby needs good physical care.

Of course feeding is his greatest pleasure in life and therefore links physical with emotional care, but your baby doesn't just need someone who'll come and feed him when he's hungry, he needs someone to come when he needs company, someone who notices when he smiles and smiles back, who hears when he "talks", listens and replies. Somebody who plays with him and shows him things, brings little bits of the world for him to see. These are the things which really matter to three month babies. These are the things which make for love.

Every baby needs at least one special person to attach himself to and more are better. It is through this first love relationship that he will learn about himself, other people and the world. It is through them that he will experience emotions and learn to cope with them. And it is through this baby love that he will become capable of more grown-up kinds of love; capable, one far-distant day, of giving children of his own the kind of devotion he now needs for himself. Babies who never have a special person, receiving adequate physical care but little emotional response, or being looked after by a succession of caretakers, often do not develop as fast or as far as their innate drive and their potential for personality allow. And the development of babies who are suddenly separated from parenting people is put at risk. But as long as your baby does have at least one special person he can make other people special too. His capacity for love is not rationed any more than yours is. The reverse is true. Love creates love.

If you and your partner are fortunate enough to be able to share your baby's care from the beginning, he will probably respond equally to each of you in total (though differently since you are different people) and his emotional life will be both richer and safer for not being vested in one person alone. That does not mean that you will get equal shares of smiles, or cooperation about stopping crying or going to sleep, on any given day, though. The baby who has the luxury of two available parents will often play favorites. Most babies start out most relaxed of all with their birth mothers – perhaps due to long familiarity with their smells, heartbeats and voices, as well as to the bliss of breastfeeding. By four or five months though, fathers, rather especially the father who has not been continually involved in a baby's routine care, may suddenly find himself singled out for favor. When he does come home, or stays home because it is a weekend, his face, his talk and his play strike the baby as fresh and interesting. Because he has not spent the day trying to fit a sufficiency of chores and sanity-preserving adult activities around the baby's needs, he may be able to offer additional social contact your baby craves.

Once that special relationship is made, sharing your time between the baby and paid outside work will not threaten it or the baby's well being provided that he continues to be – and to feel that he is – your primary concern, and that the care that fills in for yours is enthusiastic and genuinely loving. Sharing your baby's care with your partner, with other relatives or with a caregiver whom you pay to act like family, is a modern version of the way babies used to be cared for in extended families in the West, and a Western version of the way they still are cared for in much of the developing world. Don't expect those other people to keep your baby on ice for you, though. He must get on with living and loving in your absence, however much you dread him seeing his first snowfall without you or learning to love them as well. Once babies know their mothers and fathers from everybody else, they go on knowing. And once they love them best, they go on doing that too.

Many women don't want to share their babies with paid work this soon, though, because they passionately enjoy this stage of motherhood. Your baby flatters you with their special attentions, making you feel unique, beloved, and irreplaceable. They need you for everything; for adequate physical care and for emotional and intellectual care too; play, toys, help with each successive effort and opportunity to practice each tiny new accomplishment. Whatever your baby becomes able to do, he needs and will want to do it; it is up to you to make it possible for him. Yet despite all this needing, their hour-by-hour care is comparatively easy. Your baby is no longer as irrational and incomprehensible as he was when he was newborn, yet he is not awake most of the day and into everything as he will be in the second half of the year. You still get daytime periods of peace and privacy and you can still put the baby on the floor and know that your baby will be safely there when you next look.

But some women dislike it. Instead of taking pleasure in being so enjoyed and needed, they feel shut in and consumed by the baby's dependence, yearning for at least a little time when the baby needs nothing practical and nothing emotional either. The continual effort of identifying with his feelings, noticing his needs and padding his journey through the passing days makes them feel drained and once they being to feel like that, practical baby care seems easy compared with coping with an infant's loneliness or boredom.

Understanding your own importance is probably the best prevention and the most likely cure. All the vital developments of these months are waiting inside your baby. Your baby has a built-in drive to practice every aspect of being human, from making sounds, using his hands or rolling over, to eating real food or roaring with laughter. But each aspect of this growing up is also in your hands. You can help them develop and learn or you can hinder them by holding yourself aloof. You can keep your baby happy and busy and learning fast, or leave your baby to be discontented, bored and learning slowly.

If you do help your baby to learn, you and the whole family will gain because your baby will be comparatively cheerful and easy and a pleasure to have around – most of the time. If you refuse to teach your baby, trying to ration your attention, everyone will suffer and you will suffer most of all. The baby will be difficult, fretful and little pleasure to anyone. You will be unhappy because, however much you may resent the fact, your pleasure and your baby's are tied together.

If you please your baby, this happiness will please you and make it easier for you to go on. If you leave your baby miserable, this misery will depress you and make parenting more difficult. You may resent the crying at times; resent the fact that your baby needs you – again. But ignoring the crying not only condemns your baby to cry but also condemns you to listen to the crying.

So when you look to meet your baby's needs, tune in to your baby, and treat your baby as they ask to be treated, you not only do it for your baby, you also do it for yourself too. You are a family now. You sink or swim together. Loving a baby in this way is the best investment there is. It pays dividends from the very beginning and it goes on paying you returns for all the years that you have together. Your baby is, after all, a brand new human being. You are, after all, the makers and the founders of this child. As you watch and listen to your baby, think about and adjust yourselves to your baby, you are laying the foundations for a friendship that is meant to last forever."

Reprinted with kind permission from Your Baby and Child: From Birth to Age Five by Penelope Leach.

## Positive Discipline: The First Three Years

"The months leading up to the birth of a child are filled with joy, dreams, plans—and a few worries. As a caring parent, you want to start your child out in life on the proper foundation. But where do you go for the answers to such questions as: How do I communicate with an infant who doesn't understand words? How can I effectively teach boundaries to my toddler? Should I ever spank my child?

Over the years, millions of parents have come to trust Jane Nelsen's classic Positive Discipline series. These books offer a commonsense approach to child-rearing that so often is lacking in today's world. In Positive Discipline: The First Three Years, you'll learn how to use kind but firm support to raise a child who is both capable and confident. You'll find practical solutions and solid advice on how to:

- Encourage independence and exploration while providing appropriate boundaries.
- Use non-punitive methods to instill valuable social skills and positive behavior inside and outside   the home.
- Recognize when your child is ready to master the challenges of sleeping, eating, and potty training, and how to avoid the power struggles that often come with those lessons.
- Identify your child's temperament.
- Understand what the latest research in brain development tells us about raising healthy children.
- You will also learn:
  • Why punishment is never appropriate for children of any age.
  • Why any kind of time-out is not appropriate for children under the age of four, and how to create a positive time-out area "with" your four- or five-year-old that is encouraging, empowering, and teaches valuable life skills.
  • How the brain develops, and why parents often expect things of their children that are not developmentally or age appropriate -- such as sharing, apologizing, and understanding "no" the way you think they do.
  • The three most important discipline tools to use with children under the age of three.
  • Many other parenting tools that can be used with children under the age of three -- and even more that can be used with four- and five-year-olds.
  • How to get children to cooperate because they "want" to.
  • How to help your children develop the belief that, "I am capable, I can contribute in meaningful ways, and I can use my power in useful ways."
  • To remember why you had children in the first place.

All Positive Discipline parenting tools are based on kindness and firmness and at the same time they consider age and developmental appropriateness.

## Positive Discipline Guidelines

1. Misbehaving children are "discouraged children" who have mistaken ideas

on how to achieve their primary goal which is "to belong". Their mistaken ideas lead them to misbehavior. We cannot be effective unless we address the mistaken beliefs rather than just the misbehavior.

2. Use encouragement to help children feel belonging so the motivation for misbehaving will be eliminated. Celebrate each step in the direction of improvement rather than focusing on mistakes.

3. A great way to help children feel encouraged is to spend special time being with them. Many parents and teachers have noticed a dramatic change in a problem child after spending five minutes simply sharing what they both like to do for fun.

4. When tucking children into bed, ask them to share with you their saddest time during the day and their happiest time during the day. Then you share with them. You will be surprised at what you learn.

5. Have family meetings or class meetings to solve problems with cooperation and mutual respect. This is the key to creating a loving, respectful atmosphere while helping children develop self-discipline, responsibility, cooperation, and problem solving skills.

6. Give children meaningful jobs. In the name of expediency, many parents and teachers do things that children could do for themselves and one another. Children feel belonging when they know they can make a real contribution.

7. Decide together what jobs need to be done. Put them all in a jar and let each child draw out a few each week; that way no one is stuck with the same jobs all the time. Teachers can invite children to help them make class rules and list them on a chart titled, "We Decided." Children have ownership, motivation, and enthusiasm when they are included in decisions.

8. Take time for training. Make sure children understand what clean the kitchen means to you. To them it may mean simply putting the dishes in the sink. Parents and teachers may ask, "What is your understanding of what is expected?"

9. Teach and model mutual respect. One way is to be kind and firm at the same time – be kind to show respect for the child, and firm to show respect for yourself and the needs of the situation. This is difficult during conflict, so use the next guideline whenever you can.

10. Proper timing will improve your effectiveness tenfold. It does not work to deal with a problem at the time of conflict – emotions get in the way. Teach children about cooling-off periods. You or the child can go to a separate

room and do something to make you feel better – and then work on the problem with mutual respect.

11. Get rid of the idea that in order to make children do better, first you have to make them feel worse. Do you feel like doing better when you feel humiliated? This suggests a whole new look at "time-out".

12. Use Positive Time Out. Let your children help design a pleasant area with cushions, books, music and stuffed animals that will help them to feel better. Remember that children do better when they feel better. Then you can ask when they are upset, "Do you think it would help you to take some positive time out?"

13. Punishment may "work temporarily" if all you are interested in is stopping the misbehavior for "the moment". Sometimes we must be aware of what works in the short term if the long-range results are negative and create resentment, rebellion, revenge or retreat behavior in the child.

14. Teach children that mistakes are wonderful opportunities to learn. A great way to teach children that mistakes are wonderful opportunities to learn is to model this yourself by using the method of recovery after you have made a mistake. Recognize: What was the mistake. Reconcile: Be willing to say "I'm sorry, I didn't like the way I handled that." Resolve: Focus on solutions rather than blame.

15. Focus on solutions instead of consequences. Many parents and teachers try to disguise punishment by calling it a logical consequence. Get children involved in finding solutions that are related, respectful, reasonable, and helpful.

16. Make sure the message of love and respect gets through. Start with, "I care about you. I am concerned about this situation. Will you work with me on a solution?"

17. Have fun!"

Reprinted with the kind permission of Jan Nelson, Ed.D and Lynn Loft, M.A., Copyright 2006. Jan Nelson is coauthor of the bestselling Positive Discipline series, and a licensed marriage, family and child therapist. Her books have sold more than a million copies. Lynn Loft is a nationally known speaker and therapist and has coauthored many other books in the Positive Discipline series. For further information on the following books: Raising Self-Reliant Children in a Self-Indulgent World, Positive Discipline, Positive Discipline for Teenagers, Positive Discipline in the Classroom and other important parenting research go to www.positivediscipline.com.

# Conclusion

I hope you and your partner have enjoyed this guide and that you have found the information within these pages to be of value to you and your family. My heartfelt thanks go out to the love, support and guidance from the hundreds of women, aged 16 to 70, who participated in this project. I am deeply grateful for the articles from childbirth researchers from around the world that are included to assist you in the journey of creating your new family. One of my greatest joys is to hear from the mothers who have read this book and have thanked me for helping them to heal their previous birth experiences and for giving them the courage to have another baby; these women are the true heroes.

I founded the Canadian Childbirth Association to provide pregnancy, childbirth, breastfeeding and newborn care educational kits to young women and men through our existing educational system. It is imperatively important for women and men of childbearing years to be informed of the natural birth process and what they can do to create a safe and gentle labor and delivery for mother and baby.

Presently less than ten percent of new parents attend prenatal classes due to finances, time, and energy or class availability. Educating at the prenatal level is often far too late; many decisions about childbirth are made in advance of pregnancy. The time to educate is before a woman is pregnant, before fears surrounding childbirth become present. Studies show women would make better choices during childbirth if they had better information to base their decisions on.

School health programs are not complete without giving basic pre-parenting information to the students. I am convinced of the absolute importance of ensuring women have current and practical knowledge about their own bodies and their natural childbirth process. It is only through education that we will reduce the fear surrounding childbirth for all women and be able to create safe and gentle births for the tremendous benefit of all our society.

I am continuously amazed at the miracle of life and birth, most especially when I gaze into the eyes of my beautiful daughter. Let us respect this miracle of birth. A calm, gentle entry into life is the best gift we can give our children, our mothers, our fathers and our world.

Best wishes to you and to your new family,
**Gail J. Dahl**

# About The Author

Gail J. Dahl is the national best-selling author of "Pregnancy & Childbirth Secrets" and national bestselling "Pregnancy & Childbirth Tips". She is a childbirth researcher, educator and an advocate for safe and gentle childbirth. Dahl is the founder and Executive Director of the Canadian Childbirth Association and the past Vice President of CAPSAC, the Calgary Association of Parents and Professionals for Safe Alternatives in Childbirth.

Gail Dahl has created a Pregnancy & Childbirth DVD Kit that can be easily used by any teacher at any level of schooling to educate students about pregnancy, childbirth, breastfeeding and newborn care. Her aim is to dissipate the fear of childbirth through public school education so that all young women and men can participate in the planning of a safe and gentle birth for their new family.

Dahl frequently appears on television and radio and has co-hosted two pregnancy television programs. Her work encompasses the wisdom of mothers, childbirth professionals and childbirth researchers from around the world.

Gail Dahl has received the following awards for her work in women's health: YWCA Woman of Distinction Award 2000 – Education and Social Services Award, The, Woman of Vision Award 2001 for Women's Health, she has been entered into The Herstory Journal 2002 and was awarded as one of the Great Women of the 21st Century 2006.

# Acknowledgments

To the professionals; physicians, midwives, naturopaths, homeopaths, registered nurses, professional labor support people, doulas, prenatal educators and instructors, breastfeeding specialists, newborn caregivers, childbirth researchers and educators who reviewed and commented on this guide and who contributed their unique point of view, both personally and professionally, I give my heartfelt thanks.

I would also like to thank the following women for their excellent support and contributions to the project. Thanks to the others not listed who also gave of their time, ideas, and energy to help make this project happen for women.

This book has become a tapestry, brilliantly woven through, with the love that women have for one another.

| | |
|---|---|
| Abraham, Margaret | Abraham, Valerie |
| Abrahamson, Cheryl | Allyjan, Arlette |
| Anderson, Kari | Andersons, Mar |
| Apassin, Shirley | Apfield, Lisa |
| Babin, Kimberly | Balker, Jane |
| Beck, Janine | Begley, Sharon |
| Berg, Lily | Berreth, Selina |
| Bishop, Daphne | Blasetti, Karen |
| Boettcher, Monica | Boles, Franka |
| Bowen, Melanie | Brouwers, Nicole |
| Bruce, Deanna | Campbell, Jo-Anne |
| Chovancak, Beata | Colecallough, Kathleen |
| Collins, Bridget | Cohen, Nancy Wainer |
| Comito, Rosa | Cross, Maureen |
| Cuttrill, Linda | Dahl, Chelsea |
| Dahl, Kathy | Dahl, Nola |
| Dahl, Sabrina | Dahl, Sarah |
| Debiche, Dorothy | Debott, Iris |
| DeMarco, Carolyn | Devetten, Linda |
| Dinsmore, Katherine | Dobson, Rosemary |
| Dorosh, Natasha | Doucette, Dori Gallelli |
| Dubrick, Kathryn | Duffee, Sonya |
| Dusang, Tanya | Edwards, Julie |
| Eichhorst, Shelley | Eschpeter, Colleen |

Estner, Lois
Farris, Lois
Flaig, Kim
Fox, Rebecca
Galas, Ula
Gardy, Jade
Gillespie, Christine
Goer, Henci
Goulet, Laura
Grandy, Charlotte
Grant, Denise
Greene, Vanecea
Halls, Anita
Harper, Carol
Harries, Sandra
Henderson, Therese
Hernandez, Tina
Hill, Angie
Holnus, Dorothy
Huculak, Elaine
Isabella, Melanie
Janissen, Marlene
Johnson, Christie
Johnston, Marion
Jones, Louise
Kardal, Lori
Kitzinger, Sheila
Kovach, Sylvie
Lawson, Darcy
Lefebrre, Kathy
Lemke, Andy
Loewen, Michelle
Luke, Barbara
Lyon, Iris
Macdonald, Anne
Manuel, Barb
Marsh, Kim
McKeage, Wendy

Elliot, Grace
Fink, Kimberley
Fordyce, Patricia
Fraser, Bobbie
Gardy, Ernie
Gilhooly, Kathleen
Giroux, Janis
Golant, Susan
Gourley, Gwynneth
Graham, Janis
Greene, Aeriol
Griffin, Nancy
Harms, Jamie
Harper, Michelle
Helenka, Lauren
Herkert, Kimberly Ann
Hibberd, Justine
Hill, Nadia
Honard, Lynne
Hurley, Janette
Jacobsen, Gloria
Jessmaine, Cheryl
Johnston, Cheryl
Joncas, Leanne
Kabtiymer, Zenebech
Kenrick, Mariam
Kolibar, Shelley
Lamb, Lynn
Leach, Penelope
Leibel, Dee
Lindstrom, Denise
Ludington-Hoe, Susan
Luxford, Joy
MacAusland, Margaret
MacDonald, Colette
Merricks, Cathy
McKay, Margaret
McPhee, Paula

Melling, Helen
Mikkelson, Fay
Moulton, Meryl
Nagy-Cherrett, Heather
Nation, Barbara
Nightingale, Joanna
Patterson, Mrs.
Place, Kelly
Poppleton, Sharon
Priaulx, Tina
Randall, Kim
Reid, Catherine
Rod, Susan
Saint, Emilia
Sandwell, Jollean
Serhan, Nancy
Sewyl, Francine
Sinanon, Stephanie
Smythe, Angela
Spooner, Cindy
St.Pierre, Shawna
Skyllard, Rose
Taylor, Rachael
Vestrum, Tammy
Warner, Kim
Wiebe, Joy
Willson, Sharon
Winters, Staci
Young, Robin

Milne, Vivian
Morales, Karla
Mulanson, Lisa
Nason, Zoria
Nicholls, Debbie
O'Neil, Melody
Picketts, Helene
Placksin, Sally
Pratt, Jodi
Raby-Dunne, Susan
Raymond, Kitty
Rehlinger, Lucy
Rychyk, Rose
Sanche, Cynthia
Scarlett, Sheila
Sethi, Sarla
Shepard, Trish
Sinclair, Lee
Sonnenberg, Carol
Stech, Brenda
Stevens, Dave
Szrubec, Barb
Turner, Karen
Wallach, Joel
West, Joy
Williams, Delane
Wilson, Lynn
Young, Catherine

# CHILDBIRTH RESOURCE DIRECTORY

To assemble your personal health team in North America or Europe, contact your local Childbirth Association or your local Midwife Association for referrals for the best birth physicians, birth clinics, midwives, doulas, professional labor support assistants, prenatal instructors, lactation consultants, breastfeeding groups and postnatal support for your city.

Childbirth Associations and Midwife Associations are not-for-profit groups and are staffed by volunteer parents and professionals who are there to help you design the best birth for you, your partner and your baby whether you choose to have your baby at a birth centre, home or hospital.

## Professional Research Sites

The Lancet  www.thelancet.com
British Medical Journal  www.bmj.com
Medscape  www.medscape.com
Medline  www.nlm.nig.gov
American Public Health Association  www.apha.org
Risk Management Foundation (RMF) of Harvard Medical Institutions: www.rmf.harvard.edu
Society of Obstetricians and Gynecologists  www.sogc.medical.org
Canadian Institute for Health Information (CIHI):  www.cihi.ca
Multidisciplinary Collaborative Primary Maternity Care Project (MCP2): www.mcp2.ca

## Regional Sites Across the United States

Coalition for Improving Maternity Services (CIMS)  www.motherfriendly.org

American College of Nurse Midwives (ACNM)   www.acnm.org
Doulas  www.doulaworld.com
Doulas of North America (DONA)  www.DONA.org
Citizens for Midwifery  (CFM)  www.cfmidwifery.org
International Cesarean Awareness Network (ICAN) www.ican-online.org
International Childbirth Educators Association (ICEA)  www.icea.org
Midwifery Today  www.midwiferytoday.com
Midwives Alliance of North America (MANA)  www.mana.org
National Association of Childbirth Assistants (ALACE)  www.alace.org
National Association of Independent Childbearing Centers (NAICC)
www.birthcenters.org
North American Registry of Midwives (NARM)  www.narm.org

## Regional Sites Across Europe

Association for Improvements in the Maternity Services www.aims.org.uk
Caesarean Birth and Vaginal Birth after Caesarean  www.caesarean.org.uk
Home Birth Reference Site  www.homebirth.org.uk
National Childbirth Trust  www.nctpregnancyandbabycare.com
One Mother, One Midwife  www.onemotheronemidwife.org.uk
Sheila Kitzinger  www.sheilakitzinger.com
Gentlebirth  www.gentlebirth.org
Maternity and the Newborn – Royal Society of Medicine
www.motherhood.org.uk

## Regional Sites Across Canada

Alberta Association of Safe Alternative Childbirth  www.asac.ab.ca
Birth Unlimited Childbirth Association  www.birthunlimited.ca
Canadian Doulas  www.canadiandoulas.com
Doulas of Canada  www.doulasofcanada.bravehost.com
Alberta Association of Midwives (AAM)  www.albertamidwives.com
Manitoba Midwives  www.manitobamidwives.com
Midwives Association of British Colombia (MABC)  www.bcmidwives.com
Midwifery Consumer Network  www.midwiferyconsumers.org
Homebirth Association of British Columbia  www.homebirthbc.com
College of Midwives of Manitoba  www.midwives.mb.ca
Midwives Association of New Brunswick  www.manb-asfnb.ca
Association of Midwives of Newfoundland and Labrador Midwives
www.ucs.mun.ca/~pherbert

Association of Ontario Midwives (AOM)   www.aom.on.ca
Regroupement des sages-femmes du Quebec (RSFQ)   www.rsfq.org
Midwifery Education Program - Laurential University
www.midwifery.laurentian.ca
Midwifery Education Program - McMaster University www-
fhs.mcmaster.ca/midwifery
Midwifery Education Program - Ryerson University
www.ryerson.ca/midwife
Midwifery Program - University of British Columbia   www.midwifery.ubc.ca

## International Midwifery Sites
Midwives Online   www.midwivesonline.com/
Midwives Alliance of North America   www.mana.org
Royal College of Midwives (UK)   www.rcm.org.uk

## Other Related Parenting Sites
Childbirth Education -   Birthworks   www.birthworks.com
Breech Birth   www.breechbabies.com
Birthing From Within   www.birthpower.com
Bradley Method of Childbirth Education www.bradleybirth.com
Lamaze Childbirth Education   www.lamaze.org
International Childbirth Education Association   www.icea.org
International Cesarean Awareness Network   www.ican-online.org
Doulas of North America   www.dona.org
Global Birth Institute   www.globalbirth.org
Hypnobirthing   www.hypnobirthing.com
La Leche Breastfeeding Support   www.lalecheleague.org
The Breastfeeding Committee   www.breastfeedingcanada.ca
Women's Health Matters Resource Database: www.womenshealthmatters.ca
Motherstuff - Midwifery Page:
www.motherstuff.com/html/2midwifery.html/learn
Mother & Baby Wellness www.motherwellness.com
Birthwaves - Midwifery Supplies   www.birthwaves.com
Maternal Source – Childbirth Books, Videos and DVD's
www.maternalsource.com
Dr. Tom Brewer – Nutritionalist   www.blueribbonbaby.org
Compleat Mother Magazine   www.compleatmother.com
Choices Childbirth Education and Doula Services   www.birthservices.com

Clinical Hypnotherapy services for the Childbearing Year
www.midwiferyconsulting.com
Association for the Improvement of Maternity Services BC (AIMS BC)
www.aimsbc.org
The Canadian Women's Health   www.cwhn.ca
The Centre of Excellence for Women's Health   www.centres.ca
Serena – Fertility Cycles   www.serena.ca
About Pregnancy with Robin Weiss   www.pregnancy.about.com
Fetal Alcohol Syndrome   www.fetalalcohol.com
Shaken Baby Syndrome   www.shakenbaby.com
Mothering Magazine   www.mothering.com
Midwifery Today E-Magazine   www.midwiferytoday.com
Homebirth   www.homebirth.org.uk

# Bibliography

Acredolo, Linda and Susan Goodwyn. Baby Signs: How to Talk with Your Baby Before Your Baby Can Talk. Chicago. Contemporary Books, 1996.

Arms, Suzanne, Immaculate Deception II, Myth, Magic and Birth, Berkley, CA, Celestial Arts, 1996

Balaskas, Janet. The Water Birth Book, London, Thorsons Element, 2004.

Beech, Beverly Lawrence, Choosing A Waterbirth, London, AIMS 1998.

Beech, Beverley Lawrence, Ultrasound - Weighing the Propaganda, Midwifery Today, Issue 51, Autumn 1999.

Beech, Beverly Lawrence, Drugs in Pregnancy and Labor: What Effects Twenty Years Hence, Midwifery Today. Issue 50, Summer 1999.

Burch, Frances. Babysense. New York. St. Martin's Press, 1991.

Burton Goldberg Group. Alternative Medicine: The Definitive Guide. Future Medicine Publishing Inc., 1995.

Buckley, Sarah J., MD, Gentle Birth, Gentle Mothering: The Wisdom and Science of Gentle Choices in Pregnancy, Birth and Parenting, Brisbane, Australia, One Moon Press, 2005.

Carter, Jenny and Therese Duriez. With Child: Birth Through the Ages. Edinburgh. Mainstream Publishing, 1986.

Coalition for Improving Maternity Services (CIMS), Mother-Friendly Childbirth Initiative, London, England, 2007.

Coalition for Improving Maternity Services (CIMS), Problems & Hazards of Induction of Labor, London, England, 2007.

Cohen, Nancy Wainer and Lois J. Estner. Silent Knife: Cesarean Prevention and Vaginal Birth After Cesarean. New York. Bergin and Garvey, 1984.

DeMarco, Carolyn, MD. Take Charge of Your Body. Well Woman Press, 1997.

Dorey, Meryl, Why Parents Question Vaccination, Informed Voice Magazine - Your Health, Your Rights, Your Options, Australia, 2007.

England, Pam & Horowitz, Rob, Birthing From Within: An Extraordinary Guide to Childbirth Preparation, Albuquerque NM, Patera Press, 1998.

Eisenberg, Arlene, Heidi Eisenberg Murkoff, and Sandee Eisenberg Hathaway. What To Expect When You Are Expecting. New York. Workman Publishing, 2002.

Eisenberg, Arlene, Heidi Eisenberg Murkoff, and Sandee Eisenberg Hathaway. What To Eat When You Are Expecting. New York. Workman Publishing, 1986.

Eisenberg, Arlene, Heidi Eisenberg Murkoff, and Sandee Eisenberg Hathaway. What to Expect the First Year. New York. Workman Publishing, 2004.

Eisenberg, Arlene, Heidi Eisenberg Murkoff, and Sandee Eisenberg Hathaway. What to Expect the Toddler Years. New York. Workman Publishing, 2007.

Gieve, Katherine. Balancing Acts on Being a Mother. London. Virago, 1989.

Glenn, Stephen H. and Jane Nelsen EdD. Raising Self-Reliant Children in a Self-Indulgent World: Seven Building Blocks for Developing Capable Young People. Rocklin, CA. Prima Publishing, 1989.

Glenn, Stephen H. and Jane Nelsen EdD. Positive Discipline. Rocklin, CA. Prima Publishing, 1995.

Gaskin, Ina May, Ina May's Guide to Childbirth, New York, Bantam, 2003.

Gaskin, Ina May, Spiritual Midwifery, TN, The Farm Publishing, 1990.

Goer, Henci. Obstetric Myths Versus Research Realities. Westport, CT. Bergin & Garvey, 1995, The Thinking Woman's Guide to a Better Birth, Perigee, 1999.

Griffin, Nancy, MA, AAHCC, New Effective Pain Relief for Labor and Delivery, Mothering Magazine 1998.

Harper, Barbara, RN. Gentle Birth Choices. Rochester, Vermont. Healing Arts Press, 3rd Edition, 2005.

Horn, Angela, Optimum Fetal Positioning www.homebirth.org.uk. Jean Sutton and Pauline Scott, New Zealand, Birth Concepts, 'Understanding and Teaching Optimal Foetal Positioning' 2001.

Hunt, Jan, The Natural Child: Parenting from the Heart, Gabriola Island, BC New Society Publishers, 2001.

International Cesarean Awareness Network, Inc. Vaginal Birth After Cesarean, Questions and Answers, USA, 2007.

Kitzinger, Sheila, The New Pregnancy and Childbirth: Choices & Challenges, London, Dorling Kindersley, 2003, Rediscovering Birth, London, Little Brown 2000.

Kitzinger, Sheila. Breastfeeding Your Baby. New York. Alfred A. Knopf, 1989.

Kitzinger, Sheila. Homebirth: The Essential Guide to Giving Birth Outside of a Hospital. New York. Dorling Kindersley, 1991.

Kitzinger, Sheila. The Complete Book of Pregnancy & Childbirth. New York. Knopf, 1996, The Politics of Birth, London, Elsevier, 2005.

Kitzinger, Sheila. The Crying Baby. Great Britain. Penguin Books, 1990.

Klaus & Klaus. The Amazing Newborn. New York. Addison Wesley 1988.

Klaus & Klaus. Mothering The Mother: How a Doula Can Help You Have a Shorter, Easier and Healthier Birth. New York. Addison-Wesley Publishing, 1993.

Kleiman, Karen, R. NSW and Raskin, Valerie D. MD. This Isn't What I Expected: Recognizing and Recovering from Depression and Anxiety After Childbirth. New York. Bantam, 1994.

Kurcinka, Mary. Raising Your Spirited Child: A Guide for Parents Whose Child is More Intense, Sensitive, Perceptive, Persistent or Energetic. New York. Harper Collins, 1991.

Korte & Scaer. A Good Birth, A Safe Birth. New York. Bantam, 1990.

Laird, Suzanne. Choices in Childcare. Calgary. Detselig Enterprises, 1992.

Landis. Checklist for Your New Baby. New York. Berkley Book, 1993.

La Leche League. The Womanly Art of Breastfeeding. New York. New American Library, 1991.

Leach, Penelope. Your Baby and Child. New York. Addison-Wesley, 1997.

Lemay, Gloria Pushing for First-Time Mothers, Midwifery Today, Issue 55, Autumn 2000.

Leboyer, Frederick. Birth Without Violence. New York. Knopf, 1975.

Lichy, Roger & Eileen Herzberg. The Waterbirth Handbook: A Guide to the Gentle Art of Waterbirthing. Bath. Gateway Publishing, 1993.

Lieberman, Adrienne. Easing Labor Pain. Boston, Mass. Harvard Press, 1992.

Linden, Paula and Susan Gross. Taking Care of Mommy. New York. Franklin Watts, 1983.

Ludington-Hoe, Susan M., PhD with Susan Golant. Kangaroo Care: The Best You Can Do To Help Your Preterm Infant. New York. Bantam Books, 1993.

Luke, Barbara, ScD, MPH, RN, RD. Every Pregnant Woman's Guide to Preventing Premature Birth: Reducing the Sixty Proven Risks That Can Lead to Prematurity. New York. Times Books, 1995.

Machover, Ilana, Angela Drake, and Jonathon Drake. The Alexander Technique Birth Book. New York. Sterling Publishing, 1993.

McCartney, Marion CNW and Antonia VanderMeer. The Midwife's Pregnancy and Childbirth Book: Having Your Baby Your Way. New York. Henry Holt & Company, 1990.

McCracken, Leilah, Resexualizing Childbirth: A Collection of Essays, Coquitlam, BC Birthlove 2000.

Milos, Marilyn Fayre RN, Exposing the Secrets about Circumcision, 2007.

Morales, Karla and Charles B. Inlander, Take This Book To The Obstetrician With You. New York. Addison-Wesley Publishing, 1991.

Morrone, Wenda. Pregnant While You Work. New York. Berkley, 1986.

Nechas, Eileen and Denise Foley. What Do I Do Now? New York. Fireside, 1992.

Nelson, Jane, Erwin, Cheryl and Duffy, Roslyn, Positive Discipline: The First Three Years, Three Rivers Press, New York, 2003.

Nelson, Jane, and Lott, Lynn, Positive Discipline for Teenagers, Roseville, CA, Prima Publishing, 2000

Nelson, Jane, Lott, Lynn and Glenn, Stephen, Positive Discipline in the Classroom, Three Rivers Press, New York, 2000.

Odent, Michel MD. Birth Reborn. London. Souvenir, 2005, The Scientification of Love, London, Free Association Books 2001, The Caesarean, London, Free Association Books, 2004.

Panuthos, Claudia. Transformation Through Birth. Mass. Bergin & Garvey, 1984.

Pederson, Susan, Fertility Options, Avenue Magazine, Calgary, Alberta, 2006.

Pryor and Pryor. Nursing Your Baby. New York. Harper Collins Publishers, 1991.

Ridgeway, Roy. Caring for Your Unborn Child. Northamptonshire. Thorsons, 1990.

Rocissano, Lorraine and Jean Grasso Fitzpatrick. Helping Baby Talk. New York. Avon Books, 1990.

Rosen, Mortimer and Lillian Thomas. The Cesarean Myth: Choosing the Best Way to Have Your Baby. New York. Penguin Books, 1989.

Sammons, William. The Self-Calmed Baby. New York. Little Brown & Co., 1989.

Schrotenboer, Kathryn and Joan Solomon Weiss. Pregnancy Over 35. New York. Ballentine, 1985.

Sears, William MD, The Baby Book: Everything You Need to Know About Your Baby from Birth to Age Two, Boston, Little Brown, 2003.

Sears, William MD and Martha Sears RN. The Baby Book. New York. Little Brown & Co., 1993.

Simkin, Penny, Janet Whalley and Ann Keppler. Pregnancy, Childbirth and the Newborn. New York. Simon & Schuster, 1991.

Sloane, Philip, Salli Benedict and Melanie Mintzer. The Complete Pregnancy Workbook. Ontario. Key Porter Books, 1986.

Smutny, Joan, Kathleen Veenker, and Stephen Veenker. Your Gifted Child. New York. Ballentine, 1989.

Stephen, Glenn and Nelsen, Jane, Raising Self-Reliant Children in a Self-Indulgent World, Rocklin, CA, Prima Publishing, 1988.

Ulene, Art and Steven Shelov. Bringing Out the Best in Your Baby. New York. Collier Books, 1986.

Unwin, Carol Dix. Working Mothers. London. Hyman, 1989.

Verny, Thomas R. Nurturing the Unborn Child. New York, Delacorte Press, 1991.

Wagner, Marsden, MD, MS, Creating Your Birth Plan: The Definitive Guide to a Safe & Empowering Birth, Perigee Trade, USA, 2006.

Wagner, Marsden, MD, MS, Cytotec Induction and Off Label Use, Midwifery Today, Issue 67, Fall 2003.

Wagner, Marsden, Pursuing the Birth Machine: The Search for Appropriate Birth Technology, Australia, ACE Graphics, 1994.

Weiss, Robin Elise, BA, LCCE, ICCE-CPE, Repeated Miscarriage, 2006,

Weiss, Robin Elise, BA, LCCE, ICCE-CPE, Reasons to Avoid Induction of Labor, 2006, www.pregnancy.about.com.

Young, Catherine. Mother's Favorites. Toronto, NC Press, 1988.

Young, Catherine. Mother's Best Secrets. Toronto, NC Press, 1992.

# Glossary

## A

**Abruptio placentae**: a condition in which the placenta separates from the inner wall of the uterus before the baby is born. Normally the placenta does not begin separating from the uterus until after birth has occurred, but if this process occurs before or during labor, the baby's lifeline for oxygen and nutrients is cut off at the source.

**Active Birth**: a method of remaining active during labor and delivery in order to reduce pain during labor. Activity is also used to assist the baby to move into proper positioning for delivery.

**Amniocentesis**: an optional prenatal test for the removal of a sample of amniotic fluid by means of a needle inserted through the mother's abdominal wall; used for genetic and biochemical analysis of the baby. Risk to the health of the mother and baby.

**Amniotic fluid**: the liquid surrounding and protecting the baby within the amniotic sac throughout pregnancy.

**Amniotic sac**: the membrane within the uterus that contains the baby and the amniotic fluid.

## B

**Basal body temperature (BBT)**: your temperature when taken in the morning, upon awakening and before beginning activity. Used to predict ovulation.

**Bifidobacterium**: a 'healthy' bacteria, which is capable of destroying parasites, isn't actually present in mother's milk. Instead, certain carbohydrates present only in breastmilk encourage these bacteria to flourish in the baby's intestinal tract leading to a substantially reduced incidence of acute diarrhea disease.

**Breech**: position of the baby awaiting delivery in which the baby's buttocks or feet are nearest the birth canal.

## C

**Cervix**: the neck of the uterus; Pap smears are taken from the cervix.

**Cesarean section**: surgical removal of the baby through an incision into the skin of the abdomen, the underlying tissues, and the uterus.

**Chlamydia**: bacteria associated with various diseases of the eye and urogenital tract; may be transmitted by sexual contact. This is the most common infection passed from mother to baby; the baby may develop pneumonia (often a mild case) and eye infections. Although the best time to treat the mother for Chlamydia is before pregnancy, antibiotics can be administered during pregnancy to prevent infant infection. Antibiotic ointment used at birth protects the newborn from eye infection.

**Chorionic villus sampling**: an optional prenatal test in which a needle is placed through the abdomen, to the Chorionic villi, the embryonic tissue that forms the placenta, to withdraw a tissue sample for chromosomal and genetic analysis. This can only be performed after 10-12 weeks of gestation. Risk to the mother and baby.

**Clomid**: a brand name for clomiphene citrate, a synthetic hormone that stimulates the pituitary and ovulation. Another brand name is Serophene.

**Constipation**: being unable to move the bowels on a regular basis can cause the blood pressure rate to rise dangerously high in a pregnant woman.

**Complex Oligosaccharides**: the blend of these carbohydrates in breastmilk is unique. In addition to providing calories, these compounds prevent bacteria from binding to cell surfaces and can also protect against urinary tract infections.


**D**

**Delivery**: the physical expulsion of the baby by the uterus. The mother can be moved into a gravity assisted, upright position. Walking, squatting, or sitting on the toilet often helps at the time of delivery. Waiting until the urge to push develops allows her to coordinate her pushing efforts with those of her uterus. Have the woman urinate before she begins pushing. Change positions at least once every half an hour. Standing, squatting, sitting on the toilet, lying on one side, and all fours positioning can all be very effective in delivery. Avoid letting the mother lie flat on her back. Natural sensations may include backache, nausea, intense pressure on the rectum, an urge to empty the bowels, pressure, burning or stretching sensations.

The mother may want to see and touch her baby's head as it emerges from her body. This contact may renew her spirits and energy and help her focus on bringing her baby out. Avoid prolonged breath holding or prolonged pushing. Short pushes can be combined with long pushing. A mirror can help a woman to focus on tightening her pelvic floor muscles to help prevent the baby's head from moving in and out through contractions to move the delivery process along.

Encourage the woman to use low sounds and moaning to help to further release the natural opening for the baby. During a long second stage a woman needs nourishment to keep up or restore her energy level. Help her to release tension in her mouth, shoulders and legs. Keep the atmosphere calm and peaceful to assist the woman in focusing on the delivery and the eminent arrival of her baby.

Naturally occurring pain relief mechanisms, natural hormones, in the mother's body will assist the mother to relax into the sensation of contractions and stretching during the final stages of delivery. Baby needs to be placed close to the mother's breast to assist the infant with instinctual breastfeeding. Placental cord may remain attached until the delivery of the placenta to ensure the infant is able to take advantage of its natural, enriched cord blood supply and to assist the baby's first breaths. Keep mother and infant warm after childbirth.

**Diethylstilbestrol (DES)**: a synthetic, nonsteroidal estrogenic compound. Currently, it is sometimes used after sex to prevent implantation of the fertilized egg. Women whose mothers took DES during pregnancy (at a time when it was wrongly thought to prevent threatened miscarriage) can pass it along to their unborn children, causing stillbirth or birth defects. This was banned by the US FDA in 1971 for use in pregnant women. Risk to the mother and baby.

**Doula**: a doula provides emotional and physical support to the mother and father during pregnancy, labor, birth, breastfeeding and newborn care. Doulas may be called childbirth assistants, labor support professionals, birth assistants or birth companions.

**Due Date**: The estimated arrival of the baby, between 38 and 42 weeks.

**Dystocia**: difficulty in labor due to factors involving the fetus or the mother. If it cannot be resolved, delivery may have to be by cesarean section.

**E**

**Eclampsia**: the final stage of toxemia syndrome/pre-eclampsia/eclampsia. It is signaled by the occurrence of one or more convulsions. These are often preceded by spiking blood pressure, seriously increased levels of protein in the urine, and exaggerated reflex reactions, as well as severe headache, nausea or vomiting, irritability, restlessness, and twitching, upper abdominal pain, visual disturbances, drowsiness, fever, or rapid heartbeat.

**Ectopic pregnancy**: a pregnancy occurring elsewhere than in the uterus, most often in a fallopian tube. Symptoms include spasmodic cramps and pain with tenderness starting on one side and often spreading throughout the abdomen; pain may worsen on straining of the bowels, coughing, or moving. Often, brown vaginal spotting or light bleeding, intermittent or continuous, may precede pain by several days or weeks. Sometimes nausea and vomiting, dizziness or weakness, shoulder pain, and/or rectal pressure may be experienced. Getting to the hospital immediately is important. Unless the fallopian tube has irreparable damage, it is usually possible to save it, either by surgery or medication with immediate medical attention.

**Endocrine**: the system of glands that secrete hormones.

**Endometrial biopsy**: the removal of a small sample of uterine lining (endometrium) through the cervix, done for laboratory analysis between the 21st and 25th days of the menstrual cycle. Helps determine evidence of ovulation.

**Endometriosis**: a condition in which pieces of the endometrium (uterine lining) are located outside the uterus; often results in severe pain and infertility.

**Epidermal Growth Factor**: this hormone like substance is important to the growth and maturation of the linings of the baby's liver, heart, intestines, kidney, pancreas and stomach and is found in breastmilk.

**Epidural**: a local anesthetic, consisting of an anesthetic with a narcotic and/or anti-hypertensive agent, injected into the space between the outer membrane covering the spinal cord and the overlying bones of the spine. Possible side effects include hypotension, urinary retention, incontinence, paralysis of lower extremities, headache, backache, septic meningitis, slowing of labor, increased need for forceps or vacuum delivery, nerve palsies, allergic reactions, nausea, vomiting and seizures. Approximately 70% of women experience some side effects from epidurals. Effect of epidural medication on the newborn may result in a decrease in muscle tone and strength decreasing breastfeeding ability, respiratory depression, fetal malpositioning; an increase in fetal heart rate variability creating a need for forceps, vacuum, cesarean deliveries and episiotomies. Risk to the mother and baby.

**Episiotomy**: An incision used to enlarge the vaginal opening in the late stages of labor. It will make recovery longer and more painful for the woman. An episiotomy, (surgical incision) will take longer to heal than a natural tear.

**F**

**Fetal Alcohol Syndrome (FAS)**: The sum total of the damage done to the baby before birth as a direct result of the mother drinking alcohol during pregnancy. Prenatal alcohol exposure is the most common cause of mental retardation. Risk to the baby.

**Fetus**: The baby from the end of the eighth week until birth.

**Fibroid tumors**: Nonmalignant growths within the wall of the uterus that may expand during pregnancy. Occasionally, these cause problems, increasing slightly the risk of ectopic pregnancy, miscarriage, placenta previa, abruptio placenta, premature labor, premature rupture of the membranes, stalled labor, fetal malformation, and breech and other more difficult to deliver fetal positions.

**Follicle**: (mature ovarian follicle) a small sac in the ovary in which the egg develops.

**Follicular phase**: the first half of the menstrual cycle, prior to ovulation. During this phase, the follicles grow and the eggs mature until ready to be released.

**G**

**Genetic counseling**: the advice offered by experts in genetics on the detection, consequences, and risk of recurrence of chromosomal and genetic disorders.

**Gestation**: the period of fetal development in the womb from implantation to birth.

**Gestational diabetes**: carbohydrate intolerance during pregnancy that usually resolves itself after delivery. Can usually be controlled through diet and, if necessary, medication. About 3% of pregnancies are complicated by diabetes.

**Gonorrhea**: a contagious inflammation of the genitals. Can cause conjunctivitis, blindness, and serious generalized infection in the baby if delivered through an infected birth canal. Drops of silver nitrate or an antibiotic ointment can be squeezed into the eyes of the newborn at birth as an extra precaution if the mother has had gonorrhea.

**Gynecologist**: a doctor who specializes in the diseases and the routine physical care of the reproductive system of women.

**H**

**Health Danger Signals**: early contractions, leaking amniotic fluid, bleeding or spotting, fainting, seeing black spots, cramping or any marked change in the pregnancy. Contact your physician or midwife immediately.

**Hemorrhage**: profuse, life-threatening bleeding.

**Herpes**: any of several inflammatory viral diseases of the skin characterized by clusters of vesicles (blisters). Herpes is an infection that can be harmful to pregnancy. It is passed on through skin-to-skin contact. Simplex 1 is usually seen in the form of mouth sores, while simplex 2 includes sores on the genitalia. Simplex 2 can cause serious health problems or the death of a baby if the baby is vaginally delivered while the mother has active herpes on the genitals; therefore, active herpes on the genitals during labor often requires a Cesarean section. Simplex 1 can cause early health problems; people with mouth sores should therefore not be allowed to kiss your child. Active herpes can also delay infertility treatments such as in vitro fertilization.

**Hyperventilating**: the result of breathing in and out fast and furiously, this can be avoided by having the woman keep her shoulders and throat relaxed and encouraging her to breathe rhythmically.

**Hypothyroidism**: diminished production of thyroid hormone, leading to clinical manifestations of thyroid insufficiency, including low metabolic rate, tendency to gain weight, somnolence, and sometimes myxedema (severe hypothyroidism). Hypothyroidism can lead to infertility or miscarriage by disrupting the balance of hormones, especially estrogen, leading to a thin uterine lining and ovulatory dysfunction.

**I**

**Immunology**: a science that deals with the immune system.

**Implantation**: the process by which the fertilized egg attaches to the uterine lining. Usually occurs around 1 week after the egg is fertilized.

**Induction of labor**: the process, not always successful, in which labor is started by artificial means due to a pregnancy complication. Medically hastening or inducing the birth of a baby. Risk to the mother and baby.

**J**

**Jaundice**: breastfeed the baby as much as possible in the first three days to help eliminate or prevent jaundice. Colostrum, the first milk, is designed to help your baby to expel the first black, green and then yellow stools. Consult your health team if your baby has lethargy, is refusing to feed or any other unusual behaviors.

**K**

**Kegels**: pelvic floor muscles of a woman that can be exercised to help reduce urinary incontinence, to help relieve and reduce hemorrhoids, reduce pain during delivery and used to help shape and tone after childbirth.

**L**

**Labor**: the process of giving birth to a baby from when the contractions start to the baby's delivery or the time taken for this process. Labor can be reduced by the time-honored birthing traditions including walking, changing positions, rocking and even floating in water. Movement will automatically improve the efficiency of contractions, thereby shortening labor and decreasing pain. Avoiding unnecessary medical interventions during labor will decrease pain. Drinking and eating during labor can also dramatically decrease pain and increase effectiveness of contractions. All movement support rotation and alignment which assist the baby to turn and move downward through the pelvis. A professional labor coach will also decrease pain felt during labor as the laboring woman is coached into different laboring positions and techniques by the doula

**Lactoferrin**: the protein found in breastmilk that delivers iron directly to where it's needed in the intestinal lining and sequesters unnecessary iron.

**Long-Chain Polyunsaturated Fatty Acids**: These fatty acids found in breastmilk become part of the cell membranes of the infant's nervous system and are thus important to the continued development of the retina and brain. Responsible for the enhanced visual acuity of breastfed babies.

**Luteinizing hormone (LH)**: a hormone secreted by the pituitary during the entire menstrual cycle, with a peak just before ovulation. May be given therapeutically in infertility conditions. LH is the hormone that urine home-testing kits use to predict ovulation.

**Lyosozme**: an enzyme found in breastmilk. This enzyme acts like a powerful little Pac Man in the baby's digestive system. It chops up bacterial cell walls, powerfully and selectively gobbling up disease carrying bacteria.

**M**

**Midwife**: midwives are primary caregivers, meaning they care for pregnant women on their own responsibility like a physician or obstetrician.

**Meconium**: the dark greenish feces that have collected in the intestines of an unborn baby and are released shortly after birth. If the baby is under stress meconium can be expelled in the amniotic fluid. A mucus extractor ready to suck out meconium gently, before the baby's body is born and the chest has expanded to take the first breath is needed if fresh meconium is passed during the late stages of labor.

**Morning Sickness**: nausea and vomiting experienced by many pregnant women, usually in the morning and during the early months of pregnancy.


**O**

**Obstetrician**: a physician specializing in surgical delivery.

**Ovary**: the female organs that produce sex hormones and ova (eggs).

**Ovulation**: the release of a mature, unfertilized egg from the ovary.


**P**

**Pelvic inflammatory disease (PID)**: infection and inflammation of the woman's pelvic organs. Thought to be a cause of some cases of infertility.

**Perinatal doctor/perinatologist**: a doctor specializing in treating the baby and mother during pregnancy, labor, and delivery, particularly when the mother and/or baby are at a high risk for complications.

**Pitocin (oxytocin)**: a drug (given intravenously) used to induce labor.

**Placenta**: a spongy, vascular organ that supplies the baby with maternal blood and nutrients through the umbilical cord which is birthed after the baby. Left to itself the uterus will clamp down uniformly and will sheer off the placenta in one smooth sweep, but if poked and prodded it may only release in certain sections causing a postpartum hemorrhage. The placenta cannot contract, so it peels away from the lining of the uterus, usually within half an hour of the birth and slips down the vagina. The placenta must be examined to ensure all of it has been expelled. (In a lotus birth, the placenta and umbilical cord are left with the infant until the cord naturally dries, utilizing all the stored materials for the baby after childbirth.)

**Placenta previa**: a condition in which the placenta is located over the cervix, creating a risk of hemorrhage during labor and delivery. The placenta is known to migrate during the last stages of pregnancy and this condition may not appear during labor as the placenta migrates again to another location.

**Postnatal Depression**: a disorder consisting of severe depression that can affect a woman soon after giving birth.

**Pre-eclampsia**: development of hypertension (high blood pressure) with proteinuria (an excess of urinary protein) or edema (an excessive amount of fluid in the tissues), or both, due to pregnancy or the influence of a recent pregnancy; it usually occurs after the 20th week of gestation but may develop before this time in the presence of trophoblastic disease. High blood pressure can be dangerous to the mother and can lead to early induction of labor as a means of protecting the mother's life. Also called "toxemia." Pre-eclampsia may be caused by poor nutrition.

**Prenatal Visit**: planned visits with your physician or midwife to discuss your state of health during your pregnancy.

**Prenatal Class**: a series of classes taken during your pregnancy and before childbirth.

**Premature**: a baby born before 37 weeks' gestation.

**Premature Rupture of the Membranes**: a release of some of the amniotic fluid surrounding the baby. A normal occurrence in the course of labor, watch for signs of fever while monitoring mother.

**Preterm**: labor that begins between the 20th and 37th weeks of pregnancy.

**Progesterone**: a female hormone · important during pregnancy and menstruation. It is secreted by the corpus luteum to prepare the endometrium for implantation and later by the placenta during pregnancy to prevent rejection of the developing baby.

**Prolactin**: helps activate and enhance the infant's immune system and is found in breastmilk, helps to decrease the risk of ear infection in babies.

**Prolapsed Cord**: Usually a consequence of a birth intervention, in particular of rupturing the membranes artificially when the presenting part of the baby is very high which creates an obstetric emergency. Diagnosed by a marked deceleration in the fetal heart rate immediately after the artificial membrane rupture.

**Pushing Urge**: it is possible for a woman to have a baby without deliberately pushing the baby out. Keeping the mother in an upright position will assist in the baby being naturally and instinctually expelled by the uterus and the pelvic floor muscles.

## R

**Reproductive endocrinologist**: An endocrinologist specializing in reproductive disorders.

**Rhogam**: an immunization given to Rh-negative women after a miscarriage, stillbirth, or live birth to prevent production of antibodies in any Rh-positive babies they may have in future pregnancies.

**Rubella (German measles)**: a viral disease characterized by headache, fever, rash, and inflammation of the throat. Infection in a pregnant mother can damage the baby. The risks are greater the earlier in the pregnancy that the mother contracts the illness.

**S**

**Secondary infertility**: the inability of a couple to conceive after a previous successful pregnancy.

**Sexually transmitted disease (STD)**: any disease that can be transmitted by sex, such as syphilis.

**Shoulder Dystocia**: when a baby is head down, sometimes a big head is born and then there is a delay in the delivery of the shoulders. If this should occur the woman must move her positioning to release the shoulders. Hands and knees or standing position will work best in this case.

**Sialated Mucins**: combinations of carbohydrate and protein found in breastmilk with sialic acid help prevent viral diarrhea in the infant. These mucins pick up harmful viruses as they pass through the baby's intestine and transport them out.

**Sialic Acid**: important for normal cell membrane function and brain development. Breastmilk contains about ten times more sialic acid than formula does.

**Sonogram (also called ultrasound)**: a visualization of internal organs achieved by bouncing sound waves into the area to be examined (for example, a pregnant woman's abdomen). A level 1 ultrasound is usually done to approximately date a pregnancy. A level 2 ultrasound is used for more specific diagnostic purposes. Sonograms can detect a number of problems, but like all medical tests, they are not 100% perfect.

**Spina bifida**: an abnormality in the development of the spine that can cause severe neurological impairment and paralysis. Folic acid can prevent this birth defect.

**T**

**Threatened miscarriage**: an incidence in which certain symptoms, such as vaginal bleeding or severe cramping, occur during pregnancy. The symptoms may stop or may progress to a miscarriage.

**Transition Period**: During this late stage of labor most women strongly need other people to help them cope with and accept the intense contractions that are normal for this time in labor. Have the mother continue with warm baths or showers, hot towels, position changes, walking, nourishment, and frequent urination. Try other comfort measures such as cold compresses, pressure on her back, pelvic rocking, massage or stroking. Let the mother use extra pillows, a bean bag or the father to lean against for added comfort. Have her rest and relax between contractions. Help the mother stay upright and walking as long as possible. Alternate periods of activity and rest as needed. Have the mother deal with her contractions one at a time and not think about how long it has been or how long it will be.

**Toxemia**: see "pre-eclampsia."

**Toxoplasmosis**: infection by disease caused by bacteria that invades the tissues and may seriously damage the central nervous system, especially of infants. It also may be transmitted by a mother to her unborn child, resulting in abnormalities such as water on the brain (hydrocephalus), the development of jaundice shortly after birth, etc. Often found in cat feces, which is why doctors ask their pregnant patients to refrain from changing kitty litter during pregnancy.

**Trimester**: one of the 3-month periods into which a pregnancy is divided.

**Tubal pregnancy**: see "ectopic pregnancy."

**U**

**Ultrasound**: an imaging technique that uses high-frequency sound waves reflecting off internal body parts to create images, especially of the fetus in the womb for medical examination. Ultrasound does not always give an accurate representation.

**Uterus/Womb**: the female reproductive organ that contains the developing baby.

**V**

**Viability**: the ability of an infant to survive outside the womb.

**W**

**Waterbirth**: laboring and delivering in water to help reduce the pain of labor.

# Emergency Childbirth Preparation

## Labor

The length of labor can be reduced by time-honored traditions of walking, continually changing positions, rocking and using warm tubs and showers. Movement will automatically improve the efficiency of contractions, thereby shortening the labor and decreasing labor pain.

Avoiding unnecessary medical interventions during labor will also decrease pain. Drinking and eating during labor can dramatically decrease pain and increase the effectiveness of the labor contractions.

All movement that supports rotation and alignment will assist the baby to turn and move downward through the pelvis into a good position for birth.

## Transition Stage

During this later stage of labor most women strongly need others to help them cope with and accept the intense contractions that are normal for this time in labor. Have the mother continue with warm baths or showers, hot towels, position changes, walking, nourishment, and frequent urination. Try other comfort measures such as cold compresses, pressure on her back, pelvic rocking, massage or stroking.

Let the mother use extra pillows, a bean bag or the father to lean against for added comfort. Have her rest and relax between contractions. Help the mother stay upright and walking as long as possible. Alternate periods of activity and rest as needed. Have the mother deal with her contractions one at a time and not think about how long it has been or how long it will be.

## Delivery

The mother can be moved into a gravity assisted, upright position when ready for delivery. Walking, squatting, or sitting on the toilet often helps at the time of delivery. Waiting until the urge to push develops allows her to coordinate her pushing efforts with those of her uterus.

Have the woman urinate before she begins pushing. Change positions at least once every half an hour. Standing, squatting, sitting on the toilet, lying on one side, and all fours positioning can all be very effective in delivery. Avoid letting the mother lie flat on her back.

Natural, normal sensations may include backache, nausea, and intense pressure on the rectum, an urge to empty the bowels, pressure, burning or stretching sensations may also be present during the late delivery stage.

The mother may want to see and touch her baby's head as it emerges from her body. This contact with her baby may renew her spirits and energy and help her focus on bringing her baby out. Avoid prolonged breath holding or prolonged pushing during delivery.

Short pushes can be combined with long pushing for the most progress. A mirror can help a woman focus on tightening her pelvic floor muscles to help prevent the baby's head from moving in and out through contractions to move the delivery process along.

Encourage the woman to use low sounds and moaning to help to further release the birth opening for the baby. During a long second stage a woman needs nourishment to keep up or restore her energy level. Help her to release tension in her mouth, shoulders and legs. Keep the atmosphere calm and peaceful to assist the mother in focusing on the delivery and the eminent arrival of her baby.

Naturally occurring pain relief mechanisms of natural hormones in the mother's body are released with movement and will assist the mother to relax into the sensation of stronger contractions and stretching during the final stages of delivery. As the baby's head stretches the birth opening, warm oil or warm compresses can be used to ease delivery.

Upon birth the baby must be placed on the mother's breast to assist the infant with instinctual breastfeeding. The placental cord may remain attached until the delivery of the placenta to ensure the infant is able to take advantage of its natural, enriched cord blood supply and to assist the baby's first breaths.

Do not ever pull or tug on the umbilical cord. The placenta will be naturally delivered by the uterus about thirty minutes after the birth of the baby. The mother and baby must be kept in close contact for ease of breastfeeding. Immediate breastfeeding will help the uterus to contract and release the placenta easily and naturally. Keep mother and infant together and warm for at least a two hour period of time after childbirth to facilitate bonding, breastfeeding and the release of mothering hormones.

# NOTES

# NOTES